THE ANTI-INFLAMMATORY DIET
ONE-POT COOKBOOK

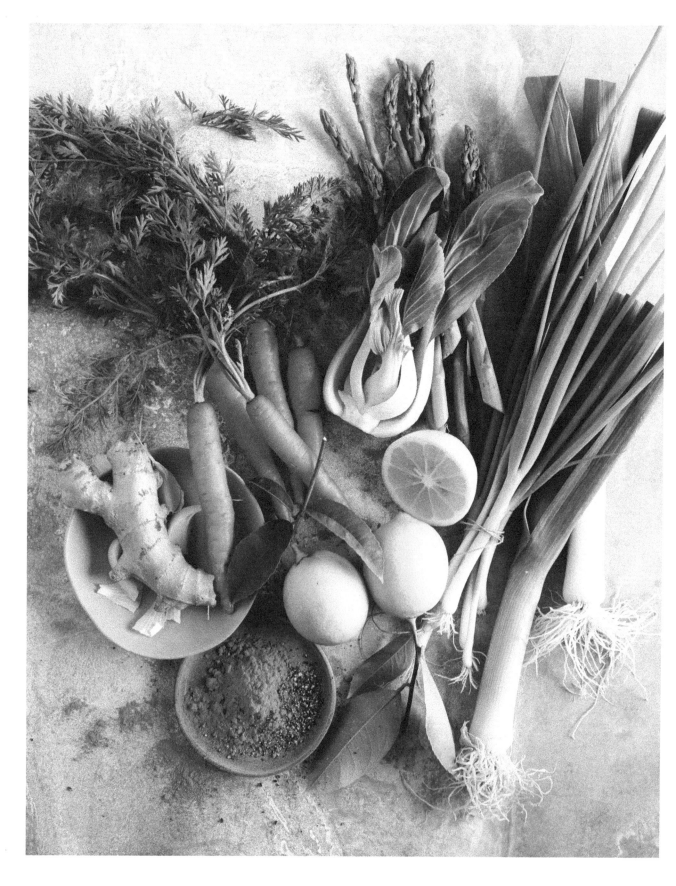

The Anti-Inflammatory Diet One-Pot Cookbook

100 Easy All-in-One Meals

Ana Reisdorf, MS, RD & Dorothy Calimeris

Photography by Jennifer Davick

ROCKRIDGE
PRESS

For general information on our other products and services or to obtain technical support, please contact our Customer Care Department within the U.S. at (866) 744-2665, or outside the U.S. at (510) 253-0500.

Rockridge Press publishes its books in a variety of electronic and print formats. Some content that appears in print may not be available in electronic books, and vice versa.

Interior and Cover Designer: Merideth Harte
Photo Art Director: Michael Hardgrove
Editor: Pam Kingsley
Production Editor: Ashley Polikoff
Photography © 2019 Jennifer Davick. Food styling by Emily Caneer.
Dorothy Calimeris photo courtesy of © Don Doblados.

ISBN: Print 978-1-64152-842-9 | eBook 978-1-64152-843-6

Dedication from Ana

This book is dedicated to Samuel and Miles,
my reasons for trying to make the world a healthier place.

Dedication from Dorothy

I dedicate this to everyone who has the courage
to explore healthier ways to eat and live.

Contents

Introduction by Ana

INFLAMMATION IS JUST A FANCY, SCIENTIFIC WORD FOR STRESS. The stress can be physical, emotional, mental, or environmental. Regardless of the source, it all boils down to the same effect. Uncontrolled stress has a significant negative impact on our bodies and our health. It is the reason why heart disease is the number one cause of death in America and why diabetes rates continue to increase. Inflammation has been linked to almost every chronic disease, from diabetes to heart disease and cancer.

As a registered dietitian nutritionist, I can see the impact of inflammation in every single person I interact with. The side effects of out-of-control stress can range from annoying, such as the inability to lose the "spare tire" around your stomach, to severe, with a diagnosis of autoimmune disease. The bottom line is that inflammation impacts everyone to some extent.

How you eat has a huge impact on inflammation. The foods you choose to eat have the power to help reduce and possibly even eliminate the symptoms and side effects of chronic stress. This book was written to provide guidance and suggestions to help you follow an anti-inflammatory diet without adding more stress to your life.

As a working mom with two young kids, I know how little time there is to prepare extensive meals, not to mention the cleanup required after. This book was designed for those who are already physically, mentally, and emotionally stressed and struggling with the side effects of inflammation. The recipes are all one-pot meals that minimize prep and cleanup to help those who are sick, exhausted, or just stretched to the limit.

No need for any appliances like a slow cooker or pressure cooker to make these recipes, just cookware you likely already own: a baking sheet, Dutch oven, soup pot, casserole dish, and salad bowl. To save you even more time, there is also a chapter dedicated to additional labor- and time-saving tips—because who wants to spend hours working in the kitchen?

The last thing anyone who is struggling with inflammation needs is additional stress. This book was developed to help you get a healthy, delicious meal on the table with minimal work. The 100 recipes provided were carefully chosen to maximize the number of anti-inflammatory ingredients while removing those ingredients that trigger inflammation.

My hope is that this book will help remove stress from your life, ease pain, and leave you feeling healthy and well nourished.

Introduction by Dorothy

IN 2015, I CREATED THE RECIPES FOR MY FIRST BOOK, *THE ANTI-INFLAMMATORY DIET & ACTION PLANS,* and I am frequently contacted by people who have purchased the book to tell me how much changing what they eat has helped them heal from stress, illness, or a lifestyle that has left them achy and depleted.

In my health-coaching practice, I have seen my clients experience significant improvement in their aches, pains, and general well-being when they adopt this style of eating. Eating an anti-inflammatory diet works, and it is my passion to make it as easy and approachable as possible.

Eating whole real food, ideally organic and locally grown, is optimal, but if cooking for yourself is intimidating and recipes are hard to follow, then it's easy to abandon your wellness plan.

This book combines all the goodness of anti-inflammatory foods with the ease of cooking at home, with simple, straightforward recipes and almost no specialized equipment. All the recipes are designed to be prepared quickly and use only one bowl, pot, or pan to prepare. Cleanup is minimal, and most recipes can be made ahead of time and packed to take to school or work. The flavors are fresh and uncomplicated, and the recipes are easily adapted to your personal tastes.

Lasting change occurs in small manageable steps, so if anti-inflammatory eating is new to you, start simply by trading processed foods for fresh foods. Initially, try only one or two recipes a week, and every week after that try a few more recipes until you have a week's worth of healthy meals that you enjoy. Although I wrote these recipes with weekday meals in mind, most are great for entertaining, whether you're bringing something to a potluck or having people over.

I love the ease of one-pot cooking, and it's how I cook most often. I hope the simplicity of this book will inspire you to look at nourishing yourself in a new way. Not only will eating whole real foods make you feel better, but also it will put the pleasure back into your meals. The vivid colors of produce, the delicious smells of food cooking, and the flavors of the ingredients and how they are combined will stimulate all your senses. Taking the time to enjoy and be present with your meal will help reduce stress, which is one of the greatest causes of inflammation. May this book be your companion on your path to wellness!

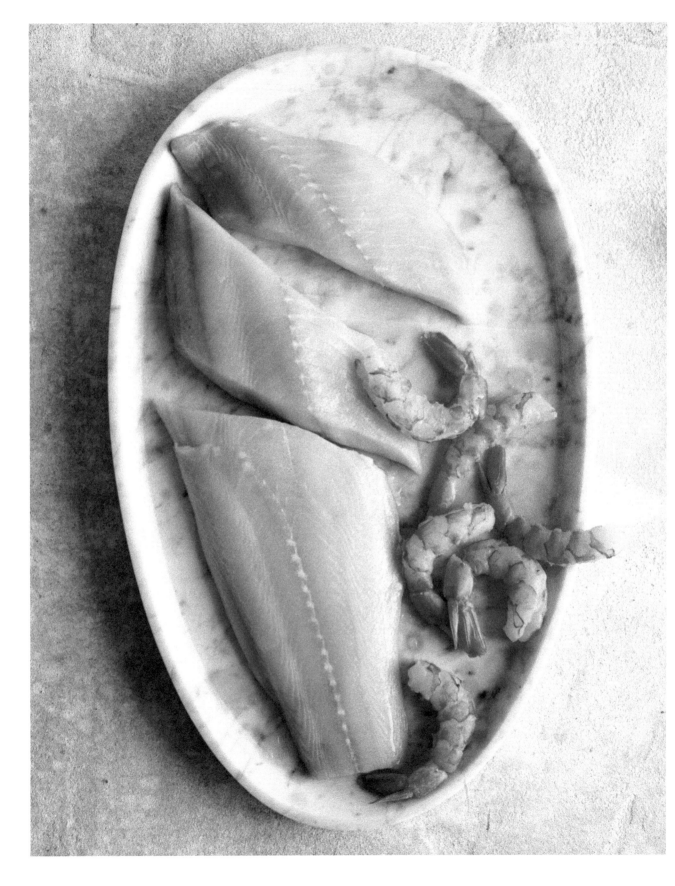

CHAPTER 1

The Anti-Inflammatory Diet

We have seen firsthand the impact that dietary changes can make on a person's health and well-being. The most impactful dietary changes are those that help promote healing from an illness or disease. This can completely change someone's life.

The first step to improving how you feel is to manage inflammation. Following an anti-inflammatory diet can help the body naturally heal and repair the damage from uncontrolled stress that leads to illness and disease.

When Inflammation Hurts

We have established that uncontrolled inflammation is the underlying cause of chronic disease. Interestingly, inflammation under normal circumstances is actually quite helpful to the body. When you have a physical injury, like a cut on your hand, the inflammatory process is triggered. The area gets red and swollen as blood rushes in. This helps immune cells and nutrients reach the area, initiating the healing process. In a few days, the cut is gone! It's really an amazing process. Once the injury is healed, the immune system should return to normal.

The problem is that many of us are struggling with low-level inflammation all the time. It never goes away. Low-level inflammation is simply an immune system that is overactive because there is no actual threat to fight. Our bodies are constantly battling an enemy that isn't really there. Scientists are not quite sure why the immune system reacts this way to our modern lifestyles. But what they do know is that when the immune system has nothing to do, it starts attacking our own organs, leading to disease.

The most extreme examples of an overactive immune system are autoimmune diseases. Conditions like lupus, rheumatoid arthritis, inflammatory bowel disease, thyroid disease, and type 1 diabetes are all a result of a severe overreaction of the immune system that leads to the destruction of organs and illness. Autoimmune diseases can be debilitating, painful, and even life-threatening, all because of an immune system gone awry.

Even without a diagnosis of autoimmune disease, you can struggle with the side effects of inflammation. Uncontrolled inflammation has been linked to:

- Cancer
- Heart disease
- High cholesterol
- Diabetes (type 1 and type 2)
- Asthma
- Central nervous system diseases, such as ALS
- Alzheimer's disease
- Gum disease
- Respiratory diseases
- Obesity
- High blood pressure

- Liver disease
- Kidney disease

As you can see, almost every organ system can be impacted by inflammation. The other problem is that inflammation doesn't just stay in one area. For example, if you have gum disease, you may also have other inflammatory conditions as well. Inflammation doesn't just limit itself to one part of the body.

What can you do about all this inflammation?

A lot, actually. Obviously, diet is a major component and the focus of this book, but lifestyle matters as well. A few ways to help lower inflammation include:

- Avoiding exposure to toxic substances, such as cigarette smoke, exhaust, or extreme pollution
- Getting enough sleep, at least 7 to 9 hours a night
- Exercising regularly
- Maintaining a healthy body weight
- Managing stress
- Spending time outdoors
- Seeking treatment for inflammatory conditions, such as gum disease or high cholesterol

In order to attack inflammation, you must target it from multiple angles. We truly believe in a holistic approach to improving one's health. No matter how perfect your diet is, it isn't going to cure anything if your stress is out of control or you sleep only four hours a night. You have to take your whole life into account if you want to reduce pain and truly live the life you want.

Our goal with this book and recipes is to give you one piece of the puzzle to help you achieve the happy, healthy life you deserve to have.

Healing Through Smart Food Choices

The first step in the battle against inflammation is to modify your diet to a more anti-inflammatory way of eating. This section outlines foods to include and foods to avoid to help you achieve this goal.

It is important to note that an "ideal" diet is highly dependent on the individual. Some foods may not work for you for various reasons, such as allergies, taste preferences, or intolerances. Only you can know your own body. These guidelines simply provide a place to start by giving you simple one-pot anti-inflammatory meals to get you feeling your best.

FOODS THAT CAN WORSEN INFLAMMATION

We might as well get the bad news out of the way: There are foods you need to avoid in order to reduce inflammation. We don't actually enjoy restricting people's diets. But we do enjoy seeing them healthy and thriving, so let's dive in.

PROCESSED MEAT

As much as meat is blamed for all the ills in the world, fresh beef, chicken, and fish are not inflammatory foods. You will see these on the "Foods to Enjoy" list. However, processed meats, such as bacon, sausage, deli meats, and hot dogs can worsen inflammation. These meats are linked to an increased risk of diseases such as diabetes, heart disease, and stroke. The reason is that they are higher in compounds called advanced glycation end products, which are known to cause inflammation. Avoid or limit processed meats as much as possible.

GRAINS

Avoid wheat and foods made from wheat. This may include breads, cereals, pasta, cakes, cookies, pies, and other desserts. The reason is that wheat contains a protein called gluten, which is a major trigger for inflammation.

Certain compounds in gluten can damage the lining of the digestive system, leading to a condition called intestinal permeability or "leaky gut." When the gut is "leaky," it allows too many food particles, microbes, and other substances to pass through without proper digestion. This causes the immune system to react to the presence of these substances, leading to dysfunction or inflammation. Avoiding foods containing gluten allows the gut to heal, a major step toward controlling inflammation.

CERTAIN FRUITS AND VEGETABLES

Most fruits and vegetables are anti-inflammatory and should be the basis of any healthy diet. The exception, for some people, are nightshades. See "The Truth About Nightshade Vegetables" (page 6) for more information on these vegetables and whether or not they should be excluded from your diet.

One thing to note about fruit: Although it is highly nutritious, it is high in sugar. Sugar sensitivity can vary from person to person. If you are sensitive to sugar, avoid eating excessive amounts of fruit. One to two servings per day is enough to meet your nutrient needs and give you a little sweet treat.

DAIRY

The evidence on dairy and inflammation is inconsistent, but dairy is a common food intolerance for many people. Lactose intolerance is one of the most common food intolerances in the world. A review of 52 studies on dairy and inflammation found that dairy was inflammatory for those who cannot tolerate it or have an allergy.

Once again, whether or not you need to avoid dairy comes down to individual tolerance. Symptoms of dairy intolerance include gas, bloating, diarrhea, or other digestive problems. These symptoms are generally more severe with liquid milk, while small amounts of cheese or yogurt can frequently be tolerated.

Since lactose intolerance is quite common, there are no recipes that include cow's dairy in this book. There are a handful of recipes using sheep's or goat's milk, as those tend to be better tolerated by most people.

CERTAIN FATS AND OILS

Canola oil, vegetable oils, trans fats, and margarine can trigger inflammation. Vegetable oils and margarine are high in omega-6 fats, which can be inflammatory at high levels, especially when they are out of balance with anti-inflammatory omega-3 fats. Canola oil should be avoided due to the way it is made. The high-heat process can cause the oil to become rancid and inflammatory.

Trans fats are man-made fats that have been removed from many foods because of their highly inflammatory properties. Trans fats are primarily found in processed foods and fried foods. By January 1, 2021, they will be completely eliminated from all foods in the United States; therefore, they will no longer be a concern.

OTHER INFLAMMATORY NO-NO'S

Foods high in sugar should also be avoided. Candy, cookies, pies, cakes, sweetened beverages, and even artificial sweeteners can trigger inflammation. Excessive sugar intake has been linked with an increased risk of inflammatory and autoimmune diseases.

Alcohol is also extremely inflammatory. Avoid alcohol of all kinds completely if you are struggling with severe inflammation.

FOODS TO ENJOY

Luckily, there are so many delicious foods to enjoy on an anti-inflammatory diet. They include:

MEAT, POULTRY, AND FISH

Fresh meats are allowed on an anti-inflammatory diet. These can include beef, poultry, pork, fish, and eggs. Protein helps you feel full and satisfied after meals, making sticking to any new eating plan a little easier.

Fish, in particular, is high in omega-3 fats, which have powerful anti-inflammatory properties. If you want even more omega-3s, choose omega-3-fortified eggs and grass-fed beef over conventionally raised.

GLUTEN-FREE GRAINS

The anti-inflammatory diet doesn't eliminate all grains. You can still enjoy oats, quinoa, millet, buckwheat, or rice, which are all naturally gluten-free. Grains are an important source of B vitamins and fiber, which help keep the digestive system healthy. Tolerance toward these grains does depend on the individual, so you may choose to avoid them if they don't work for you.

THE TRUTH ABOUT NIGHTSHADE VEGETABLES

If you search the internet for "inflammatory foods" you will likely come across nightshade vegetables on that list. Nightshades are vegetables from the *Solanum* genus. Included are tomatoes, bell peppers, eggplants, hot peppers, and goji berries, amongst others. These vegetables contain a toxic plant compound called solanine, which the plants use to defend themselves against consumption by insects. Although this compound is toxic and inflammatory, the amount in most of these vegetables is pretty minimal. Most people actually won't have inflammation after eating these vegetables, many of which are high in important nutrients, such as vitamin C.

That being said, these vegetables were left out of the recipes in the book, since some people with inflammatory conditions do react to them. The reaction may be due to food intolerances, not the solanine itself. They can always be added back in if you are not sensitive to them, because they are loaded with lots of nutrition.

MOST VEGETABLES AND FRUITS

All vegetables and fruits are allowed on the anti-inflammatory diet. (See the previous page for nightshades exceptions.) We include legumes and beans in this section as well. Plants are loaded with fiber, potassium, folate, and other important nutrients for health. They are also an incredible source of vitamins with antioxidant and anti-inflammatory properties, such as vitamins A and C. Plants are a major source of phytonutrients, or anti-inflammatory plant compounds. Fruits and vegetables should make up the majority of your diet, since they pack a major anti-inflammatory punch.

CERTAIN FATS AND OILS

Focus on monounsaturated fats, such as avocado oil and olive oil, to reduce inflammation. Small amounts of real butter or coconut oil are also fine.

Nuts, seeds, olives, and avocados all contain healthy fats and can be enjoyed on an anti-inflammatory diet.

OTHER GOOD-FOR-YOU FOODS

In addition to the foods mentioned previously, you can add flavor to your food with any herbs and spices you wish. Turmeric, cinnamon, and ginger are particularly anti-inflammatory.

Green and black tea can be a great warm beverage to kick off your morning. Coffee should be enjoyed based on individual tolerance.

Sweeten foods and drinks with small quantities of honey or maple syrup.

Include fermented foods, such as kombucha or kimchi, to support healthy digestion.

Although red wine does contain some anti-inflammatory properties, alcohol is highly inflammatory. If you are struggling with severe inflammation, you should probably avoid drinking any alcohol.

FOOD GUIDE FOR THE INFLAMMATORY DIET

FOODS TO INCLUDE	FOODS TO AVOID
All herbs and spices, particularly ginger, turmeric, cinnamon	Artificial sweeteners
All vegetables except nightshades (see page 6)	Canola oil
Avocados	Dairy (milk, cheese, yogurt)
Butter	Fried foods
Coconut oil	Margarine
Dark chocolate	Nightshade vegetables (tomatoes, white potatoes, eggplant, peppers, goji berries)
Eggs	Processed meats (bacon, sausage, deli meats, hot dogs)
Fermented foods like kimchi, kombucha	Refined carbohydrates (breakfast cereals, desserts)
Fish (especially wild-caught salmon, sardines, mackerel, anchovies, herring)	Soda and other sugar-sweetened beverages
Fruit, especially berries	Sugar and candy
Gluten-free grains (buckwheat, millet, oats, quinoa, rice, wild rice)	Vegetable oils
Gluten-free pasta	Wheat (bread, pasta, wheat-based cereals)
Grass-fed beef	
Honey, maple syrup	
Legumes (beans and lentils)	
Onion family (garlic, scallions, onions, shallots)	
Nuts and seeds	
Olive oil	
Poultry	
Soy products, including tofu	
Sweet potatoes	
Tea, green and black	

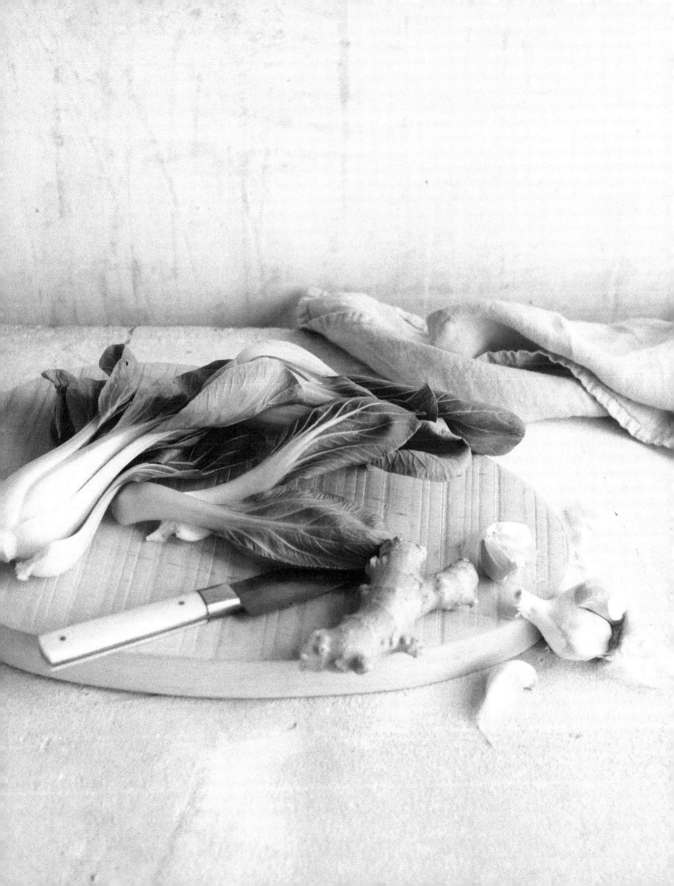

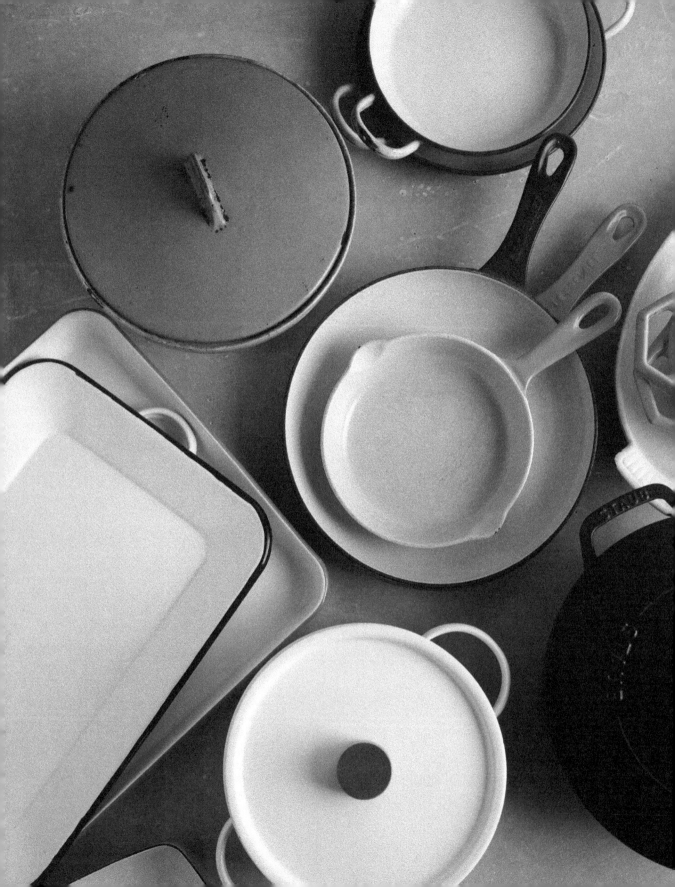

CHAPTER 2

The Anti-Inflammatory One-Pot Kitchen

Now that you know what to eat, you are ready to get to cooking. As promised, you don't need to buy any special equipment for the recipes in this book, but there are a few things you do want have on hand to make meal prep as easy and fast as possible.

Equipping Your One-Pot Kitchen

The recipes in this book call for several different types of "one-pots." Use whichever you have on hand, but if you are in the market for new kitchen equipment, here are a few suggestions for what to look for.

LARGE SALAD BOWL

Salad bowls can be made out of glass, plastic, or wood. Since you won't be heating it up, the material really depends on your personal preference. Plastic is usually the lightest and easiest to clean, so if you are struggling with an autoimmune disease or other inflammatory condition, you might choose a large plastic bowl.

SOUP POT OR LARGE SAUCEPAN

The size of the soup pot you choose will depend on how much soup or stew you need to make. Most of the recipes in this book are based on four servings, but you may have to double the recipe if you have a large family. A 6- or 12-quart pot will work for most people. Choose a lightweight material if you are struggling with pain or inflammation, to make the pan easy to get on and off the stove.

ADAPT WHAT YOU HAVE

We don't want you to feel that you have to have every piece of kitchen equipment mentioned to be successful in making these recipes. We tried to limit the recommended equipment as much as possible because we don't like having too many useless things in our kitchen either. For example, the stir-fry recipes don't call for a wok, because you can easily stir-fry in a large skillet.

There is definitely some flexibility here—if you don't have a sheet pan, you can use an uncovered oven-safe skillet. Or a Dutch oven makes for an awesome casserole dish. If the Dutch oven is just too heavy for you to use, you can easily substitute a covered skillet or large saucepan instead, so you can still enjoy the recipes in that section.

DUTCH OVEN

A Dutch oven is like a large saucepan, but is thicker and heavier. It is usually made of cast iron and has a thick, heavy lid. A 6-quart Dutch oven should be adequate for most recipes. They can vary greatly in price, anywhere from $50 to $300. Choose the best you can afford.

CASSEROLE DISH

Casserole dishes are usually made of glass, porcelain, stoneware, or cast iron. Each has different benefits and disperses the heat differently. The most cost-effective is glass. It is also see-through, making it easy to know when the dish is ready. The recipes in this book mostly call for an 8-inch, square casserole dish or baking dish.

BAKING SHEET

You will need a large rimmed baking sheet for many recipes in this book (you can also use a half sheet pan, a favorite among bakers). Baking sheets are quite versatile and can be used for a variety of dishes. However, if you don't have a baking sheet, you don't need to buy one. You can use a casserole dish or an ovenproof skillet for the same effect.

SKILLET

A skillet is a very versatile piece of kitchen equipment. It can be used to sauté, sear, and stir-fry. Choose a large skillet, since you will be preparing a whole meal with it, between 10 and 12 inches in diameter. Skillets come in a variety of materials, such as cast iron, stainless steel, or nonstick. Cast iron can be heavy and does require some additional care. If you want a nonstick option, look for those lined with ceramic, which tend to be safer for the environment than other materials and will withstand heat better.

Labor-Saving Strategies

We recognize that many who will be using this book are experiencing pain, discomfort, or fatigue of some kind. Inflammation is exhausting! The last thing you want to be doing is spending hours cooking dinner. That's why we want these recipes to be as easy as possible. We have also made an effort to limit the number of ingredients and prep time required. But there are always ways to cut back on time in the kitchen even further. Here are a few of our favorites:

INVEST IN A FOOD PROCESSOR

A food processor that slices, chops, and dices can save you a lot of time in the kitchen. There are many reliable, inexpensive models available that will do almost all of the slicing and dicing in half the time. Or if you don't want to invest in an electric food processor, consider a mini-chop that you can use to mince garlic, onions, and fresh herbs to help save time on prep.

PREP IN BATCHES

Preparing your food in batches is one of the best time-saving techniques. On Sunday (or before your week begins), wash and dice all your vegetables at once. Bag them separately in individual portions, and place them in the refrigerator or freezer. They will be cut up and ready to go when you need them, so you don't waste time on busy weeknights.

USE HEALTHY CONVENIENCE FOODS

These days, most grocery stores have a wide variety of healthy "convenience" foods, from diced and chopped vegetables to fully peeled winter squash, prewashed greens, and ready-to-serve frozen vegetables. In the meat section, you will find precooked rotisserie chicken, cubed meats, and even pre-marinated meats (although you need to check the ingredients on these). There is no reason why you can't use these types of foods to make life a bit easier.

LOVE YOUR LEFTOVERS

Always using your leftovers for other meals can help you save time and money. Leftovers make for an awesome lunch. After dinner, pack them into grab-and-go containers so they are ready for the next day. If a dish can be frozen (which is indicated on the recipes), you can always store a bank of single-servings in the freezer for meals on crazy weeknights, when you don't have the time to prepare anything.

OUR FAVORITE SUPERMARKET CONVENIENCE FOODS

> **Rotisserie chicken.** Makes for a quick weekday lunch, or can be shredded into soups or salad for added protein. (Check the ingredients in the seasonings, since they may include sugar.)
> **Pre-marinated meats.** For nights when we can't even think about what to make, these are quick and easy to prepare. (Check the ingredients in the marinade, since they may include sugar and soy sauce, which contains gluten.)
> **Pre-made kabobs.** Someone else has already taken care of prepping the meat and vegetables; now all you have to do is cook them.
> **Already peeled or cooked shrimp.** Peeling shrimp can be such a fiddly task; spend a little extra money and buy them already peeled. Already cooked shrimp are a great addition to a dinner salad.
> **Prewashed greens.** No need to spend the extra step to wash or slice again.
> **Cubed winter squash.** Cutting and peeling a raw squash can be tough, so why do it?
> **Pineapple slices.** Peeling and cutting a pineapple can be cumbersome, so let someone else handle it.
> **Watermelon cubes.** Watermelon can also be hard to cut; pre-cut allows you to enjoy watermelon without all the work.
> **Frozen vegetable "mixes."** Makes it easy to sneak a ton of vegetables into various dishes with little prep.
> **Mashed avocado.** Avocados always go bad before we eat them. They tend to last a bit longer mashed and in a prepackaged container.
> **Pre-portioned nuts.** Nuts are a great healthy snack; pre-portioned helps you take them on the go.

ORGANIZE YOUR KITCHEN FOR YOUR CONVENIENCE

How you organize your kitchen can help make cooking faster and easier as well. Try storing heavier cookware such as cast-iron pans in a place that doesn't require stooping and lifting. Keep like items together, so they are easy to find. Consider putting often-used ingredients on the counter or in a cabinet where they will be readily accessible for when you need them.

BUY TOOLS THAT WORK FOR YOU

As we mentioned, you don't need to buy anything to make these recipes. But some kitchen gadgets do make food prep a bit easier. Here are a few you may consider:

- Electric can opener
- Electric jar opener
- Glass storage containers
- Slow cooker (and liners for the slow cooker, for easy cleanup)
- Garlic press
- Meat thermometer
- Bendable cutting boards
- Spiral vegetable slicer (spiralizer)
- Mandoline

IMMERSION BLENDER

We particularly want to single out this nifty tool. It allows you to purée soups (and much more) right in the pot, making it a perfect fit for the one-pot style of cooking. No more having to carefully transfer hot soup to an upright blender to purée in batches, then transfer back to the pot for a quick warm-up. The immersion blender is a lightweight, inexpensive, and very useful tool to add to your labor-saving arsenal. Several recipes in this book call for it.

About the Recipes

Throughout the recipe section you will see various labels to help you determine which recipes best meet your individual dietary requirements. Here is a bit more detail on what they mean:

Dairy: Although products made with cow's milk are not included, we did include products made from goat's and sheep's milk. Butter is also used in a few recipes but could be substituted with a vegan plant-based margarine like Earth Balance® if you are trying to completely avoid cow products. The recipes that include these types of ingredients are labeled as Dairy.

Nuts: This means that the recipe contains peanuts or tree nuts.

Seafood/Shellfish: This indicates that the recipe contains one of these ingredients.

Vegan: Vegan means the recipe contains no animal products at all.

Vegetarian: Vegetarian recipes may contain the types of dairy mentioned earlier, as well as other foods like eggs and honey.

All the recipes also have a Tips section. This section offers additional information about the recipe, substitutions for ingredients, cooking tips and techniques, and storage suggestions.

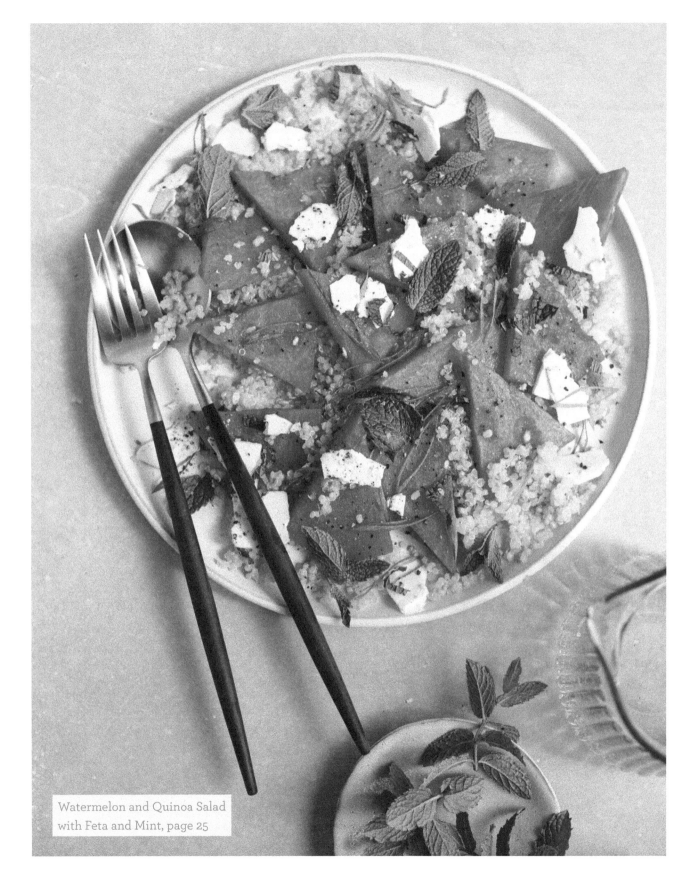

Watermelon and Quinoa Salad
with Feta and Mint, page 25

CHAPTER 3

Super Salads

I t's easy to make a one-pot or one-bowl salad that's satisfying and substantial. The salad can be created in the same pan that the vegetables were roasted in. Homemade dressing is much healthier than most store-bought brands, which are made with inferior oils and loaded with sugars, thickeners, and fillers, all of which can lead to increased inflammation in the body. These salads are dressed with simple ingredients which bring out the natural goodness. Keeping basic ingredients on hand like bagged organic greens, avocados, scallions, roasted chicken, extra-virgin olive oil, and apple cider vinegar allow you to create an anti-inflammatory meal in minutes.

LENTIL AND SPINACH SALAD WITH BUTTERNUT SQUASH

SERVES 4 / PREP TIME: 15 MINUTES / COOK TIME: 20 MINUTES

Once the butternut squash is cooked, this satisfying salad can be assembled in a matter of minutes. Lentils are high in protein and have iron and fiber. Serve this salad as a warm side dish, or eat cold or at room temperature when brown-bagging it the next day.

2 cups peeled butternut squash cut into 1-inch dice

¼ cup extra-virgin olive oil

1 teaspoon salt, divided

1 (15-ounce) can cooked lentils, drained and rinsed

4 cups baby spinach

¼ cup finely chopped red onion

¼ cup chopped walnuts (optional)

2 tablespoons freshly squeezed lemon juice

1 tablespoon finely chopped fresh sage

¼ teaspoon freshly ground black pepper

1. Preheat the oven to 400°F.

2. In a 9-by-13-inch baking dish, toss together the squash, oil, and ½ teaspoon of salt.

3. Transfer the casserole dish to the oven and roast until the squash is tender, for about 20 minutes. Remove from the oven; if serving cold, let cool before continuing with the recipe.

4. Add the lentils, spinach, onion, walnuts (if using), lemon juice, sage, remaining ½ teaspoon of salt, and the pepper, mix well, and serve.

TIPS: *Some markets sell already-cooked butternut squash and chopped red onions in the produce section, which makes this meal ready in minutes. You can store the salad, covered, in the refrigerator for several days. If you're sensitive to nuts, pumpkin seeds are a good alternative for the walnuts.*

PER SERVING Calories: 239; Total Fat: 13g; Total Carbohydrates: 25g; Sugar: 4g; Fiber: 8g; Protein: 9g; Sodium: 611mg

WHITE BEAN AND BASIL SALAD WITH SHAVED ZUCCHINI

SERVES 4 / PREP TIME: 10 MINUTES

Creamy white beans are the perfect counterpart to the shaved zucchini. Instead of pesto, which contains dairy, this recipe uses finely chopped basil and minced garlic for great Italian flavor.

¼ cup extra-virgin olive oil

¼ cup freshly squeezed lemon juice

¼ cup finely chopped fresh basil

1 garlic clove, minced

2 large zucchini, shaved with a vegetable peeler

1 (15½-ounce) can white beans, drained and rinsed

¼ cup thinly sliced scallions, both white and green parts

1 teaspoon salt

¼ teaspoon freshly ground black pepper

1. In a large bowl, combine the oil, lemon juice, basil, and garlic. Use a wooden spoon to mash the ingredients together to release the flavor in the basil and garlic.

2. Add the zucchini, beans, scallions, salt, and pepper and gently mix the ingredients, being careful to not mash the beans, and serve.

TIPS: *Shaving the zucchini sounds fancier than it is! Trim both ends of the zucchini, and use a vegetable peeler to make long thin slices. The crunchy thin slices make for a nice contrast to the soft beans. Some markets sell spiralized zucchini; you can use that instead, if you like. Store the salad, covered, in the refrigerator for several days.*

PER SERVING Calories: 269; Total Fat: 14g; Total Carbohydrates: 30g; Sugar: 4g; Fiber: 12g; Protein: 10g; Sodium: 601mg

CURRY-ROASTED CAULIFLOWER AND CHICKPEA SALAD

SERVES 4 / PREP TIME: 15 MINUTES / COOK TIME: 15 MINUTES

Even people who think they don't like cauliflower love it roasted. Most curry powders contain many anti-inflammatory spices like turmeric, cumin, and fenugreek. The chickpeas add protein and fiber, creating a complete meal.

2 cups cauliflower florets

¼ cup melted coconut oil or extra-virgin olive oil

1½ teaspoons curry powder

1 teaspoon salt

3 cups romaine lettuce cut across into 1-inch ribbons

1 (15-ounce) can chickpeas, drained and rinsed

2 tablespoons freshly squeezed lime juice

2 tablespoons chopped fresh cilantro

1 tablespoon extra-virgin olive oil

¼ teaspoon freshly ground black pepper

1. Preheat the oven to 400°F.

2. In a 9-by-13-inch baking dish, toss together the cauliflower, coconut oil, curry powder, and salt until well mixed.

3. Transfer the dish to the oven, and roast until tender, for about 15 minutes. Remove from the oven and let cool to room temperature.

4. Add the lettuce, chickpeas, lime juice, cilantro, olive oil, and pepper, toss to combine, and serve.

TIPS: *Toasted slivered almonds and shredded coconut are good additions to this salad. This salad can be made ahead of time without the lettuce and stored, covered, for several days, in the refrigerator. Add the lettuce right before serving.*

PER SERVING Calories: 275; Total Fat: 19g; Total Carbohydrates: 23g; Sugar: 5g; Fiber: 6g; Protein: 7g; Sodium: 603mg

QUINOA AND BRUSSELS SPROUT SLAW WITH BLUEBERRIES

SERVES 4 / PREP TIME: 10 MINUTES / COOK TIME: 25 MINUTES

Quinoa is gluten-free and high in protein and fiber. It cooks quickly and is easy to make in a large batch to have on hand, ready to use. Some markets sell cooked quinoa in the frozen section, making it even easier to enjoy. Shredding Brussels sprouts and eating them raw is a good way to get even the most anti–Brussels sprouts eater to try them.

1 cup quinoa

1 teaspoon salt

12 ounces Brussels sprouts, trimmed and thinly sliced

¼ cup finely chopped red onion

¼ cup extra-virgin olive oil

1 tablespoon apple cider vinegar

1 cup blueberries

1 teaspoon finely chopped fresh sage

¼ cup toasted sliced almonds (optional; see Tips, right)

1. In a large pot, combine the quinoa, 2 cups of water, and salt. Bring to a boil, reduce the heat to a simmer, and cook, partially covered, until all the water has been absorbed, for about 20 minutes. Remove from the heat.

2. Add the Brussels sprouts and onion to the warm quinoa (this will slightly soften the vegetables). Let cool to room temperature.

3. Add the oil, vinegar, blueberries, sage, and almonds (if using). Toss to combine, and serve at room temperature, or chill for several hours to serve cold.

TIPS: *If using frozen cooked quinoa, use 3 cups cooked quinoa. You can also shred the Brussels sprouts by using the slicing disk of a food processor. Toasting almonds is easy and adds a lot of flavor. Place the almonds on a small baking sheet, and transfer to a 375°F oven (or toaster oven); toast until lightly browned, for 5 to 8 minutes.*

PER SERVING Calories: 326; Total Fat: 16g; Total Carbohydrates: 41g; Sugar: 6g; Fiber: 7g; Protein: 9g; Sodium: 606mg

ROASTED WINTER VEGETABLE AND CHICKPEA SALAD

SERVES 4 / PREP TIME: 15 MINUTES / COOK TIME: 20 MINUTES

If your market sells roasted vegetables in the produce department or salad bar, load up! This salad can be enjoyed as an entrée or do double duty as a side dish. The acorn squash is unpeeled in this recipe, so be sure to wash it before you slice it.

1 small acorn squash, seeded and thinly sliced

1 cup thinly sliced carrots

½ cup thinly sliced parsnips

½ small red onion, thinly sliced

3 tablespoons extra-virgin olive oil

1 garlic clove, minced

1 teaspoon salt

¼ teaspoon freshly ground black pepper

1 (15-ounce) can chickpeas, drained and rinsed

2 cups baby arugula

1 tablespoon apple cider vinegar

1. Preheat the oven to 400°F.

2. In a 9-by-13-inch casserole dish, toss together the squash, carrots, parsnips, onion, oil, garlic, salt, and pepper until well mixed.

3. Transfer the dish to the oven, and roast until the vegetables are golden brown and tender, 15 to 20 minutes. Remove from the oven and let cool to room temperature.

4. Add the chickpeas, arugula, and vinegar, toss to combine, and serve.

TIPS: *This salad will keep for several days, covered, in the refrigerator; add the arugula shortly before serving. Baby spinach can be substituted for the arugula.*

PER SERVING Calories: 266; Total Fat: 12g; Total Carbohydrates: 35g; Sugar: 6g; Fiber: 8g; Protein: 7g; Sodium: 613mg

WATERMELON AND QUINOA SALAD WITH FETA AND MINT

SERVES 4 / PREP TIME: 10 MINUTES / COOK TIME: 25 MINUTES

This salad screams summer! The quinoa adds protein and fiber, and the watermelon is sweet and juicy and a delicious counterpart to the creamy feta. Since most markets sell cut watermelon, this salad is a breeze to create.

1 cup quinoa

1 teaspoon salt

¼ cup extra-virgin olive oil

2 tablespoons freshly squeezed lemon juice

2 cups seeded watermelon cut into ½-inch dice

1 scallion, both white and green parts, thinly sliced

½ cup crumbled sheep's or goat's milk feta cheese

¼ cup finely chopped fresh mint

¼ teaspoon freshly ground black pepper

1. In a large pot, combine the quinoa, 2 cups of water, and salt. Bring to a boil, reduce the heat to a simmer, and cook, partially covered, until all the water has been absorbed, about 20 minutes. Remove from the heat, let cool to room temperature, and fluff with a fork.

2. Add the oil and lemon juice and mix well.

3. Add the watermelon and scallion, and gently mix until just combined.

4. Sprinkle the cheese, mint, and pepper over the salad and serve.

TIPS: *If using cooked quinoa, use 3 cups. This salad is best eaten shortly after it's been made but can be stored, covered, in the refrigerator for 24 hours.*

PER SERVING Calories: 473; Total Fat: 29g; Total Carbohydrates: 36g; Sugar: 4g; Fiber: 4g; Protein: 19g; Sodium: 1189mg

CHIPOTLE AND SWEET POTATO SALAD WITH RED CABBAGE, BLACK BEANS, AND CILANTRO

SERVES 4 / PREP TIME: 10 MINUTES / COOK TIME: 20 MINUTES

Here roasted sweet potatoes contrast with the crunch of red cabbage. The black beans add protein, and the cilantro complements the smokiness of the chipotle powder. Many markets sell roasted sweet potatoes in their produce area or salad bar, which makes the prep time even shorter.

2 cups peeled sweet potatoes cut into ½-inch dice

½ small red onion, finely chopped

¼ cup extra-virgin olive oil

1 teaspoon chipotle chile powder

1 teaspoon salt

¼ teaspoon freshly ground black pepper

2 cups shredded red cabbage

1 (15-ounce) can black beans, drained and rinsed

2 tablespoons chopped fresh cilantro

1 tablespoon apple cider vinegar

1. Preheat the oven to 400°F.

2. In a 9-by-13-inch baking dish, toss together the sweet potatoes, onion, oil, chili powder, salt, and pepper until well mixed.

3. Transfer the dish to the oven and roast until the sweet potatoes are tender and lightly browned, about 20 minutes. Remove from the oven and let cool to room temperature.

4. Add the cabbage, beans, cilantro, and vinegar, toss to combine, and serve.

TIPS: *Most markets sell bags of shredded cabbage. If shredded red cabbage isn't available, a coleslaw blend will do. This salad can be stored, covered, in the refrigerator for several days.*

PER SERVING Calories: 251; Total Fat: 13g; Total Carbohydrates: 28g; Sugar: 4g; Fiber: 8g; Protein: 7g; Sodium: 623mg

JICAMA AND BLACK BEAN SALAD WITH BROWN RICE AND SALSA

SERVES 4 / PREP TIME: 10 MINUTES/ COOK TIME: 50 MINUTES

Most premade salsas contain tomatoes, which are nightshades and best avoided when eating an anti-inflammatory diet. This dish has all the flavors of salsa without tomatoes, and it makes for a great burrito filling, too. Just add mashed avocados and pack it into gluten-free tortillas.

1 cup medium- or long-grain brown rice

5 tablespoons extra-virgin olive oil, divided

2 teaspoons salt, divided

1 (15-ounce) can black beans, drained and rinsed

1 small jicama, peeled and cut into ¼-inch dice

¼ cup finely chopped fresh cilantro

¼ cup freshly squeezed lime juice

2 scallions, both white and green parts, thinly sliced

1 small jalapeño pepper, seeded and minced

¼ teaspoon freshly ground black pepper

1. In a large pot, combine the rice, 2 cups of water, 1 tablespoon of oil, and 1 teaspoon of salt. Bring to a boil, reduce the heat to a simmer, cover, and cook until the rice is tender, 40 to 45 minutes. Remove from the heat, let cool to room temperature, and fluff with a fork.

2. Add the beans, jicama, cilantro, lime juice, scallions, jalapeño pepper, remaining 4 tablespoons of oil, remaining 1 teaspoon of salt, and the pepper, and mix well. Serve at room temperature, or chill for several hours to serve cold.

TIPS: *Brown rice typically takes 40 to 45 minutes to cook; if time allows, soaking the rice in water overnight and draining it will shorten the time to 30 minutes. Or use the cooked frozen brown rice available in many markets. If using frozen brown rice, use 3 cups of cooked rice. This salad will keep, covered, in the refrigerator for several days.*

PER SERVING Calories: 449; Total Fat: 19g; Total Carbohydrates: 61g; Sugar: 2g; Fiber: 12g; Protein: 10g; Sodium: 1175mg

MEDITERRANEAN BROWN RICE SALAD WITH CHICKEN AND MINT

SERVES 4 / PREP TIME: 10 MINUTES / COOK TIME: 50 MINUTES

Brown rice is less processed than white rice, which makes it higher in B vitamins and magnesium. The nutty flavor enhances the roast chicken, and the scallions, mint, and feta create the Mediterranean flavors.

1 cup medium- or long-grain brown rice

5 tablespoons extra-virgin olive oil, divided

1 teaspoon salt

1 large zucchini, cut into ¼-inch dice

2 cups shredded rotisserie chicken

2 cups baby spinach

¼ cup freshly squeezed lemon juice

2 scallions, both white and green parts, thinly sliced

2 tablespoons chopped fresh mint

½ cup crumbled sheep's or goat's milk feta cheese

1. In a large pot, combine the rice, 2 cups of water, 1 tablespoon of oil, and the salt. Bring to a boil, reduce the heat to a simmer, cover, and cook until the rice is tender, for 40 to 45 minutes. Remove from the heat, let cool to room temperature, and fluff with a fork.

2. Add the zucchini, chicken, spinach, lemon juice, remaining 4 tablespoons of olive oil, the scallions, and mint and mix well.

3. Sprinkle with the cheese and serve.

TIPS: *Cow's milk can be hard to digest, but many people can tolerate sheep's or goat's milk products. Sheep's or goat's milk feta isn't as readily available as cow's milk feta but can be found at gourmet markets or farmers' markets. This salad will keep, covered, in the refrigerator for several days.*

PER SERVING Calories: 674; Total Fat: 39g; Total Carbohydrates: 43g; Sugar: 2g; Fiber: 3g; Protein: 41g; Sodium: 1401mg

ROASTED CHICKEN AND KALE SALAD WITH WHITE BEANS

SERVES 4 / PREP TIME: 10 MINUTES

This salad utilizes many convenience products: rotisserie chicken, bagged kale, and canned white beans. The nutrient-dense kale and beans increase the fiber. Omitting the chicken makes this a quick vegan salad.

4 cups baby kale

¼ cup extra-virgin olive oil

3 tablespoons
red-wine vinegar

1 teaspoon salt

¼ teaspoon freshly ground
black pepper

2 cups shredded
rotisserie chicken

1 (15-ounce) can white
beans, drained
and rinsed

¼ cup finely chopped
red onion

¼ cup coarsely chopped
walnuts (optional)

1. In a large bowl, using your hands, mix the kale with the oil, vinegar, salt, and pepper, massaging it into the leaves to soften them.

2. Add the chicken, beans, and onion and mix to combine.

3. Sprinkle with the walnuts (if using) and serve.

TIPS: *If available in your market, baby kale is best for uncooked kale dishes, since the leaves are more tender. The walnuts can be omitted, or any other nut can be used. If sensitive to nuts, pumpkin seeds are a good alternative. This salad can be stored, covered, in the refrigerator for several days.*

PER SERVING Calories: 348; Total Fat: 15g; Total Carbohydrates: 26g; Sugar: 1g; Fiber: 8g; Protein: 28g; Sodium: 655mg

CRUNCHY VIETNAMESE CHICKEN SALAD

SERVES 4 / PREP TIME: 15 MINUTES

This family favorite utilizes rotisserie chicken from your local market. When choosing a rotisserie chicken, choose one that is seasoned only with salt and pepper, as other spice mixes or marinades may contain sugars and unhealthy oils.

⅓ cup extra-virgin olive oil

2 tablespoons freshly squeezed lime juice

1 tablespoon distilled white vinegar

1 tablespoon fish sauce

1½ teaspoons honey

½ teaspoon minced garlic

4 cups shredded green cabbage

1 cup shredded carrots

½ small red onion, thinly sliced

2 tablespoons finely chopped fresh cilantro

2 tablespoons finely chopped fresh mint

½ serrano pepper, seeded and thinly sliced (optional)

2 cups shredded rotisserie chicken

3 tablespoons coarsely chopped peanuts (optional)

1. In a large bowl, whisk together the oil, lime juice, vinegar, fish sauce, honey, and garlic until blended.

2. Add the cabbage, carrots, onion, cilantro, mint, and serrano pepper (if using) and combine well.

3. Top the salad with the chicken, sprinkle with the peanuts (if using), and serve.

TIPS: *This salad is at its crunchiest best when eaten shortly after it has been made, but will keep for 24 hours, covered, in the refrigerator. Add the peanuts shortly before eating. Omit the chicken and fish sauce for a vegetarian version.*

PER SERVING Calories: 297; Total Fat: 19g; Total Carbohydrates: 11g; Sugar: 7g; Fiber: 3g; Protein: 22g; Sodium: 425mg

ROMAINE AND SMOKED SALMON SALAD WITH CUCUMBER AND RED ONION

SERVES 4 / PREP TIME: 15 MINUTES

This elegant salad is put together in minutes. The sweet creaminess of coconut milk yogurt is a good contrast to the smoky saltiness of the smoked salmon. This is a wonderful breakfast or brunch salad.

1 cup plain coconut
milk yogurt

1 tablespoon finely
chopped fresh chives

1 teaspoon Dijon mustard

½ teaspoon salt

¼ teaspoon freshly ground
black pepper

4 cups romaine hearts
cut across into
1-inch ribbons

1 cup thinly sliced
English cucumber

¼ cup thinly sliced
red onion

1 ripe avocado, pitted,
peeled, and thinly sliced

8 ounces smoked salmon,
thinly sliced

1. To make the dressing, in a large bowl, whisk together the yogurt, chives, mustard, salt, and pepper until smooth.

2. Add the romaine, cucumber, and onion and mix until the salad is well coated with the dressing.

3. Arrange the avocado and smoked salmon on top of the greens and serve.

TIPS: *Once made, this salad should be eaten immediately. To save time, the vegetables can be prepped and the dressing made ahead of time and stored, covered, in the refrigerator overnight.*

PER SERVING Calories: 164; Total Fat: 10g; Total Carbohydrates: 8g; Sugar: 2g; Fiber: 4g; Protein: 12g; Sodium: 1469mg

GARLICKY ROMAINE AND TUNA SALAD

SERVES 4 / PREP TIME: 15 MINUTES

This recipe utilizes the flavors of a Caesar salad but keeps within the guidelines of anti-inflammatory eating. Canned tuna and romaine hearts make this a quick and easy meal.

1 garlic clove, minced

1 teaspoon salt

¼ cup extra-virgin olive oil

1 teaspoon Dijon mustard

¼ teaspoon freshly ground black pepper

3 romaine hearts, cut into 1-inch pieces

3 (5-ounce) cans water-packed tuna, drained

½ English cucumber, thinly sliced

2 scallions, both white and green parts, thinly sliced

1 ripe avocado, pitted, peeled, and cut into ½-inch dice

½ cup grated sheep's milk pecorino cheese

1. In a large bowl, combine the garlic and salt and use a wooden spoon to mash them together to make a paste.

2. To make the dressing, add the oil, mustard, and pepper to the paste, and mix well.

3. Add the romaine, tuna, cucumber, and scallions and mix until the salad is well coated with the dressing.

4. Top with the avocado, then the cheese, and serve.

TIPS: *Anchovies can be substituted for the tuna for an even more authentic Caesar taste; since anchovies have a robust flavor, 10 ounces are enough to serve four people. This salad should be eaten within 24 hours of being made.*

PER SERVING Calories: 360; Total Fat: 26g; Total Carbohydrates: 7g; Sugar: 1g; Fiber: 4g; Protein: 25g; Sodium: 873mg

SHRIMP AND FENNEL SALAD WITH SPINACH

SERVES 4 / PREP TIME: 10 MINUTES, PLUS MARINATING TIME

The mildly licorice-like flavor of fennel pairs well with the sweet delicate flavor of shrimp. Fennel aids digestion and is high in antioxidants and a good source of fiber.

¼ cup extra-virgin olive oil

¼ cup freshly squeezed orange juice

1 tablespoon honey

1 teaspoon minced or grated orange zest

1 teaspoon salt

¼ teaspoon freshly ground black pepper

1 pound cooked peeled shrimp, thawed if necessary

1 cup shaved fennel bulb

2 scallions, both white and green parts, thinly sliced

4 cups baby spinach

1. To make the dressing, in a large bowl, whisk together the oil, orange juice, honey, orange zest, salt, and pepper until smooth.

2. Add the shrimp, fennel, and scallions, and toss until evenly coated with the dressing. Set aside for the flavors to develop, about 30 minutes.

3. When ready to serve, add the spinach, toss to combine well and coat with the dressing, and serve.

TIPS: *The best way to shave fennel is either with the thin slicing disk on a food processor or by using a mandoline. If you don't have either, you can use finely chopped fennel instead. Frozen shrimp may release a lot of liquid after it's thawed, so drain it before adding to the salad. This salad can be stored, covered, in the refrigerator for 24 hours; add the spinach shortly before serving.*

PER SERVING Calories: 264; Total Fat: 15g; Total Carbohydrates: 9g; Sugar: 6g; Fiber: 2g; Protein: 26g; Sodium: 1018mg

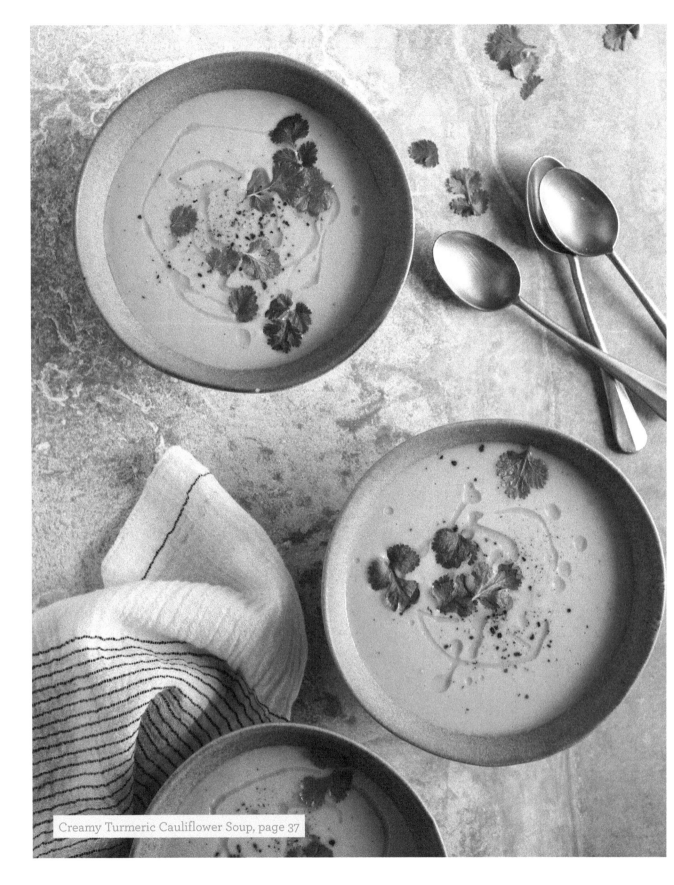
Creamy Turmeric Cauliflower Soup, page 37

CHAPTER 4

Satisfying Soups

Warm and soothing, soups are one of the best ways to make the most out of an anti-inflammatory meal plan. Simmering vegetables in water or broth creates a health elixir perfumed with all the ingredients in the pot. Soups typically last for days in the refrigerator and even longer in the freezer, making them an ideal choice for a busy life. If possible, use bone broth, which has many healing properties. For example, it can provide collagen, which may help with joint stiffness. If you are vegan or vegetarian, you can still experience the healing properties of soup by enjoying the broth that is created while making the soup.

FENNEL AND PEAR SOUP

SERVES 4 / PREP TIME: 15 MINUTES / COOK TIME: 20 MINUTES

Pears are rich in flavonoids, antioxidants, and fiber, and both pears and fennel aid in digestion. This soup can be enjoyed hot or cold and dressed up with a dollop of sheep's milk ricotta and toasted almonds if you like.

2 tablespoons extra-virgin olive oil

4 pears, cored and cut into ½-inch dice

2 fennel bulbs, trimmed and cut into ½-inch dice

2 shallots, halved

4 cups vegetable broth

¼ cup freshly squeezed lemon juice

¼ cup honey

1 teaspoon salt

¼ teaspoon freshly ground black pepper

⅛ teaspoon ground nutmeg

1 teaspoon finely chopped fresh tarragon

1. In a large pot, heat the oil over high heat.

2. Add the pears, fennel, and shallots, and sauté until the pears and fennel just begin to brown, about 5 minutes.

3. Add the broth, and bring to a boil.

4. Reduce the heat to a simmer, and cook, stirring occasionally, until the fennel is tender, 5 to 8 minutes.

5. Stir in the lemon juice, honey, salt, pepper, and nutmeg.

6. Using an immersion blender, purée the soup in the pot until smooth.

7. Sprinkle with the tarragon and serve.

TIPS: *For best results, the pears should be a tad underripe. If you'd like a creamier soup, you can add ¼ cup coconut milk or almond milk. Store the soup, covered, in the refrigerator for up to 5 days, or freeze for longer.*

PER SERVING Calories: 328; Total Fat: 9g; Total Carbohydrates: 60g; Sugar: 39g; Fiber: 10g; Protein: 7g; Sodium: 1413mg

CREAMY TURMERIC CAULIFLOWER SOUP

SERVES 4 / PREP TIME: 10 MINUTES / COOK TIME: 15 MINUTES

Turmeric is the darling of the anti-inflammatory spices. For best absorption by the body, turmeric should be combined with pepper. This soup gets its creamy texture from coconut milk, but other nondairy milk can be used instead.

2 tablespoons extra-virgin olive oil or coconut oil

1 leek, white part only, thinly sliced

3 cups cauliflower florets

1 garlic clove, peeled

1 (1¼-inch) piece fresh ginger, peeled and sliced

1½ teaspoons turmeric

½ teaspoon salt

¼ teaspoon freshly ground black pepper

¼ teaspoon ground cumin

3 cups vegetable broth

1 cup full-fat coconut milk

¼ cup finely chopped fresh cilantro

1. In a large pot, heat the oil over high heat.

2. Add the leek, and sauté until it just begins to brown, 3 to 4 minutes.

3. Add the cauliflower, garlic, ginger, turmeric, salt, pepper, and cumin and sauté to lightly toast the spices, 1 to 2 minutes.

4. Add the broth and bring to a boil.

5. Reduce the heat to a simmer and cook until the cauliflower is tender, about 5 minutes.

6. Using an immersion blender, purée the soup in the pot until smooth.

7. Stir in the coconut milk and cilantro, heat through, and serve.

TIPS: *Many markets sell cauliflower florets in the produce department. Store this soup, covered, in the refrigerator for up to a week, or freeze for several months.*

PER SERVING Calories: 264; Total Fat: 23g; Total Carbohydrates: 12g; Sugar: 5g; Fiber: 4g; Protein: 7g; Sodium: 900mg

"EAT YOUR GREENS" SOUP

SERVES 4 / PREP TIME: 10 MINUTES / COOK TIME: 20 MINUTES

If a green smoothie is not your thing, you may enjoy this soup instead.
All the goodness of greens is sweetened by the cooking process. This
recipe uses kale, Swiss chard, and mustard greens, but any combination of
greens works.

¼ cup extra-virgin olive oil

2 leeks, white parts only,
   thinly sliced

1 fennel bulb, trimmed and
   thinly sliced

1 garlic clove, peeled

1 bunch Swiss chard,
   coarsely chopped

4 cups coarsely
   chopped kale

4 cups coarsely chopped
   mustard greens

3 cups vegetable broth

2 tablespoons apple
   cider vinegar

1 teaspoon salt

¼ teaspoon freshly ground
   black pepper

¼ cup chopped
   cashews (optional)

1. In a large pot, heat the oil over high heat.

2. Add the leeks, fennel, and garlic and sauté until softened, for about 5 minutes.

3. Add the Swiss chard, kale, and mustard greens and sauté until the greens wilt, 2 to 3 minutes.

4. Add the broth and bring to a boil.

5. Reduce the heat to a simmer and cook until the vegetables are completely soft and tender, about 5 minutes.

6. Stir in the vinegar, salt, pepper, and cashews (if using).

7. Using an immersion blender, purée the soup in the pot until smooth and serve.

TIPS: *This soup makes for a great base soup to which to add all kinds of wonderful things, like cooked chicken, fish, or beans. Store, covered, for up to a week in the refrigerator, or freeze for several months.*

PER SERVING Calories: 238; Total Fat: 14g; Total Carbohydrates: 22g; Sugar: 4g; Fiber: 6g; Protein: 9g; Sodium: 1294mg

SWEET POTATO AND CORN SOUP

SERVES 4 / PREP TIME: 10 MINUTES / COOK TIME: 20 MINUTES

Sweet potatoes, mushrooms, and corn are family favorites. We've added broccoli and zucchini for extra nutrition.

¼ cup extra-virgin olive oil or coconut oil

1 medium zucchini, cut into ¼-inch dice

1 cup broccoli florets

1 cup thinly sliced mushrooms

1 small onion, cut into ¼-inch dice

4 cups vegetable broth

2 cups peeled sweet potatoes cut into ¼-inch dice

1 cup frozen corn kernels

1 cup coconut milk or almond milk

2 tablespoons finely chopped fresh flat-leaf parsley

1 teaspoon salt

¼ teaspoon freshly ground black pepper

1. In a large pot, heat the oil over high heat.

2. Add the zucchini, broccoli, mushrooms, and onion and sauté until softened, 5 to 8 minutes.

3. Add the broth and sweet potatoes and bring to a boil.

4. Reduce the heat to a simmer and cook until the sweet potatoes are tender, 5 to 7 minutes.

5. Add the corn, coconut milk, parsley, salt, and pepper. Cook over low heat until the corn is heated through and serve.

TIPS: *You can substitute any vegetables of your choice in this recipe; you can also add cooked shrimp, chicken, or beans for a more substantial soup. Store, covered, in the refrigerator for several days, or freeze for several months.*

PER SERVING Calories: 402; Total Fat: 29g; Total Carbohydrates: 31g; Sugar: 9g; Fiber: 6g; Protein: 10g; Sodium: 1406mg

CHICKPEA CURRY SOUP

SERVES 4 / PREP TIME: 10 MINUTES / COOK TIME: 25 MINUTES

The fun thing about curry soup is you can use any seasonal vegetables or protein you like. Curry blends are a powerhouse of anti-inflammatory spices. The base for this soup is butternut squash and apple, which complements the buttery flavor of chickpeas.

¼ cup extra-virgin olive oil or coconut oil

1 medium onion, finely chopped

2 garlic cloves, sliced

1 large Granny Smith apple, cored, peeled, and cut into ¼-inch dice

2 teaspoons curry powder

1 teaspoon salt

3 cups peeled butternut squash cut into ½-inch dice

3 cups vegetable broth

1 cup full-fat coconut milk

1 (15-ounce) can chickpeas, drained and rinsed

2 tablespoons finely chopped fresh cilantro

1. In a large pot, heat the oil over high heat.

2. Add the onion and garlic and sauté until the onion begins to brown, 6 to 8 minutes.

3. Add the apple, curry powder, and salt and sauté to toast the curry powder, 1 to 2 minutes.

4. Add the squash and broth and bring to a boil.

5. Reduce the heat to a simmer and cook until the squash is tender, about 10 minutes.

6. Stir in the coconut milk.

7. Using an immersion blender, purée the soup in the pot until smooth.

8. Stir in the chickpeas and cilantro, heat through for 1 to 2 minutes, and serve.

TIPS: *Chopped nuts and coconut are good toppings for this soup. Store this soup, covered, in the refrigerator for up to 5 days, or freeze for several months.*

PER SERVING Calories: 469; Total Fat: 30g; Total Carbohydrates: 45g; Sugar: 14g; Fiber: 10g; Protein: 12g; Sodium: 1174mg

ONION, KALE, AND WHITE BEAN SOUP

SERVES 4 / PREP TIME: 15 MINUTES / COOK TIME: 25 MINUTES

This soup is greater than the sum of its parts. The onion is caramelized, then simmered with kale in vegetable broth to bring out the sweetness in the kale. If you'd like to add dairy, a shower of grated sheep's milk pecorino is a delicious topping for this soup.

¼ cup extra-virgin olive oil

1 large onion, thinly sliced

2 garlic cloves, thinly sliced

1 teaspoon salt

¼ teaspoon freshly ground black pepper

⅛ teaspoon red pepper flakes (optional)

3 cups stemmed kale leaves cut into ½-inch pieces

4 cups vegetable broth

1 (15½-ounce) can white beans, drained and rinsed

1 teaspoon finely chopped fresh rosemary

1. In a large pot, heat the oil over high heat.

2. Reduce the heat to medium, and add the onion, garlic, salt, pepper, and red pepper flakes (if using). Sauté until the onion is golden, about 10 minutes.

3. Add the kale, and sauté until wilted, 1 to 2 minutes.

4. Add the broth and bring to a boil.

5. Reduce the heat to simmer, and cook until the kale is soft, about 5 minutes.

6. Add the beans and rosemary. Cook until the beans are warmed through, 2 to 3 minutes, and serve.

TIPS: *This soup can also be made with Swiss chard or spinach instead of kale. Store, covered, in the refrigerator for up to a week, or freeze for several months.*

PER SERVING Calories: 285; Total Fat: 15g; Total Carbohydrates: 28g; Sugar: 3g; Fiber: 9g; Protein: 13g; Sodium: 1368mg

BROWN RICE AND SHIITAKE MISO SOUP WITH SCALLIONS

SERVES 4 / PREP TIME: 10 MINUTES / COOK TIME: 45 MINUTES

Shiitake mushrooms have many healthy properties, including boosting immunity and heart health. They have a rich savory flavor which enriches the cooking liquid. Sesame oil and ginger give this soup its depth of flavor.

2 tablespoons sesame oil

1 cup thinly sliced shiitake mushroom caps

1 garlic clove, minced

1 (1½-inch) piece fresh ginger, peeled and sliced

1 cup medium-grain brown rice

½ teaspoon salt

1 tablespoon white miso

2 scallions, both white and green parts, thinly sliced

2 tablespoons finely chopped fresh cilantro

1. In a large pot, heat the oil over medium-high heat.

2. Add the mushrooms, garlic, and ginger and sauté until the mushrooms begin to soften, about 5 minutes.

3. Add the rice and stir to evenly coat with the oil.

4. Add 2 cups of water and salt and bring to a boil.

5. Reduce the heat to a simmer and cook until the rice is tender, 30 to 40 minutes.

6. Use a little of the soup broth to soften the miso, then stir it into the pot until well blended.

7. Stir in the scallions and cilantro and serve.

TIPS: *If using frozen, cooked brown rice, use 3 cups of brown rice in this recipe. Miso, a fermented soy product, comes in many varieties. This recipe uses white miso for its delicate flavor, but any type of miso will work well. Store this soup, covered, in the refrigerator for up to 5 days, or freeze for several months.*

PER SERVING Calories: 265; Total Fat: 8g; Total Carbohydrates: 43g; Sugar: 2g; Fiber: 3g; Protein: 5g; Sodium: 456mg

GARLIC AND LENTIL SOUP

SERVES 4 / PREP TIME: 15 MINUTES / COOK TIME: 15 MINUTES

A classic combination with a twist, this soup includes cinnamon and orange zest. Lentils are a nutrition powerhouse, high in protein and fiber. Using canned lentils shortens the cooking time. If you're in the mood for dairy, crumbled sheep's milk feta is a delicious addition to this soup.

2 tablespoons extra-virgin
olive oil

2 medium carrots,
thinly sliced

1 small white onion, cut into
¼-inch dice

2 garlic cloves, thinly sliced

1 teaspoon
ground cinnamon

1 teaspoon salt

¼ teaspoon freshly ground
black pepper

3 cups vegetable broth

1 (15-ounce) can lentils,
drained and rinsed

1 tablespoon minced or
grated orange zest

¼ cup chopped
walnuts (optional)

2 tablespoons finely
chopped fresh
flat-leaf parsley

1. In a large pot, heat the oil over high heat.

2. Add the carrots, onion, and garlic and sauté until softened, 5 to 7 minutes.

3. Add the cinnamon, salt, and pepper and stir to evenly coat the vegetables, 1 to 2 minutes.

4. Add the broth and bring to a boil.

5. Reduce the heat to a simmer, add the lentils, and cook until they are heated through, about 1 minute.

6. Stir in the orange zest and serve, sprinkled with the walnuts (if using) and parsley.

TIPS: *It's easy to double this recipe and freeze a batch to be enjoyed on a day when you're short on time. Store, covered, in the refrigerator for up to 5 days, or freeze for several months.*

PER SERVING Calories: 201; Total Fat: 8g; Total Carbohydrates: 22g; Sugar: 4g; Fiber: 8g; Protein: 11g; Sodium: 1178mg

ITALIAN SUMMER SQUASH SOUP

SERVES 4 / PREP TIME: 10 MINUTES / COOK TIME: 15 MINUTES

The zucchini is shredded in this soup, so it cooks in minutes. Use a combination of green zucchini and yellow squash for a riot of color. Many stores carry spiralized zucchini, which will work just as well. With basil and pine nuts, this is summer in a bowl. A crumble of goat cheese and a drizzle of olive oil is a delicious optional garnish.

3 tablespoons extra-virgin olive oil

1 small red onion, thinly sliced

1 garlic clove, minced

1 cup shredded zucchini

1 cup shredded yellow squash

½ cup shredded carrot

3 cups vegetable broth

1 teaspoon salt

2 tablespoons finely chopped fresh basil

1 tablespoon finely chopped fresh chives

2 tablespoons pine nuts

1. In a large pot, heat the oil over high heat.

2. Add the onion and garlic and sauté until softened, 5 to 7 minutes.

3. Add the zucchini, yellow squash, and carrot and sauté until softened, 1 to 2 minutes.

4. Add the broth and salt and bring to a boil.

5. Reduce the heat to a simmer and cook until the vegetables are soft, 1 to 2 minutes.

6. Stir in the basil and chives and serve, sprinkled with the pine nuts.

TIPS: *The easiest way to shred the vegetables is to use a food processor. Otherwise, a handheld box grater works well. You can make a winter version of this using shredded winter squash or root vegetables. Store, covered, in the refrigerator for several days, or freeze for several months.*

PER SERVING Calories: 172; Total Fat: 15g; Total Carbohydrates: 6g; Sugar: 3g; Fiber: 2g; Protein: 5g; Sodium: 1170mg

CHICKEN AND GLUTEN-FREE NOODLE SOUP

SERVES 4 / PREP TIME: 10 MINUTES / COOK TIME: 25 MINUTES

No need to forgo one of life's most soothing soups because you're avoiding gluten. There are many varieties of gluten-free pastas available now. We used penne in this recipe, but feel free to use your favorite shape of pasta.

¼ cup extra-virgin olive oil

3 celery stalks, cut into
¼-inch slices

2 medium carrots, cut into
¼-inch dice

1 small onion, cut into
¼-inch dice

1 fresh rosemary sprig

4 cups chicken broth

8 ounces gluten-free penne

1 teaspoon salt

¼ teaspoon freshly ground
black pepper

2 cups diced rotisserie
chicken

¼ cup finely chopped fresh
flat-leaf parsley

1. In a large pot, heat the oil over high heat.

2. Add the celery, carrots, onion, and rosemary and sauté until softened, 5 to 7 minutes.

3. Add the broth, penne, salt, and pepper and bring to a boil.

4. Reduce the heat to a simmer and cook until the penne is tender, 8 to 10 minutes.

5. Remove and discard the rosemary sprig, and add the chicken and parsley.

6. Reduce the heat to low. Cook until the chicken is warmed through, about 5 minutes, and serve.

TIPS: *If planning on reheating this soup, it's better to slightly undercook the pasta so that it doesn't end up getting mushy. Store, covered, in the refrigerator for several days, or freeze for several months.*

PER SERVING Calories: 485; Total Fat: 18g; Total Carbohydrates: 47g; Sugar: 4g; Fiber: 7g; Protein: 33g; Sodium: 1423mg

LEEK, CHICKEN, AND SPINACH SOUP

SERVES 4 / PREP TIME: 10 MINUTES / COOK TIME: 15 MINUTES

Using rotisserie chicken and bagged spinach makes this a super-fast and easy soup. Lemon zest brightens it up.

3 tablespoons unsalted butter

2 leeks, white parts only, thinly sliced

4 cups baby spinach

4 cups chicken broth

1 teaspoon salt

¼ teaspoon freshly ground black pepper

2 cups shredded rotisserie chicken

1 tablespoon thinly sliced fresh chives

2 teaspoons grated or minced lemon zest

1. In a large pot, melt the butter over high heat.

2. Add the leeks and sauté until softened and beginning to brown, 3 to 5 minutes.

3. Add the spinach, broth, salt, and pepper and bring to a boil.

4. Reduce the heat to a simmer and cook until the spinach wilts, 1 to 2 minutes.

5. Add the chicken and cook until warmed through, 1 to 2 minutes.

6. Sprinkle with the chives and lemon zest and serve.

TIPS: *If you can't find leeks, shallots or onions can be substituted. Store, covered, in the refrigerator for up to 5 days, or freeze for several months.*

PER SERVING Calories: 256; Total Fat: 12g; Total Carbohydrates: 9g; Sugar: 3g; Fiber: 2g; Protein: 27g; Sodium: 1483mg

SAFFRON AND SALMON SOUP

SERVES 4 / PREP TIME: 10 MINUTES / COOK TIME: 20 MINUTES

This soup is a type of bouillabaisse: a brothy soup, golden with saffron and studded with chunks of salmon. Saffron is rich in antioxidants, and salmon is rich in omega-3 fats—both help brain function. If you prefer, you can substitute saffron with ½ teaspoon turmeric. Traditionally this is served with aioli, an emulsion of olive oil and eggs, studded with minced raw garlic.

¼ cup extra-virgin olive oil

2 leeks, white parts only, thinly sliced

2 medium carrots, thinly sliced

2 garlic cloves, thinly sliced

4 cups vegetable broth

1 pound skinless salmon fillets, cut into 1-inch pieces

1 teaspoon salt

¼ teaspoon freshly ground black pepper

¼ teaspoon saffron threads

2 cups baby spinach

½ cup dry white wine

2 tablespoons chopped scallions, both white and green parts

2 tablespoons finely chopped fresh flat-leaf parsley

1. In a large pot, heat the oil over high heat.

2. Add the leeks, carrots, and garlic and sauté until softened, 5 to 7 minutes.

3. Add the broth and bring to a boil.

4. Reduce the heat to a simmer and add the salmon, salt, pepper, and saffron. Cook until the salmon is cooked through, about 8 minutes.

5. Add the spinach, wine, scallions, and parsley and cook until the spinach has wilted, 1 to 2 minutes, and serve.

TIPS: *Because of the salmon, this soup should be eaten within 48 hours of cooking. The salmon can be replaced with cod, shrimp, or a combination of seafood.*

PER SERVING Calories: 418; Total Fat: 26g; Total Carbohydrates: 13g; Sugar: 4g; Fiber: 2g; Protein: 29g; Sodium: 1455mg

BUTTERNUT SQUASH SOUP WITH SHRIMP

SERVES 4 / PREP TIME: 10 MINUTES / COOK TIME: 20 MINUTES

This chunky soup is really almost a chowder. With pre-cut butternut squash and cooked shrimp available in most markets, it's ready in minutes.

3 tablespoons
unsalted butter

1 small red onion,
finely chopped

1 garlic clove, sliced

1 teaspoon turmeric

1 teaspoon salt

¼ teaspoon freshly ground
black pepper

3 cups vegetable broth

2 cups peeled butternut
squash cut into
¼-inch dice

1 pound cooked peeled
shrimp, thawed
if necessary

1 cup unsweetened
almond milk or other
nondairy milk

¼ cup slivered
almonds (optional)

2 tablespoons finely
chopped fresh
flat-leaf parsley

2 teaspoons grated or
minced lemon zest

1. In a large pot, melt the butter over high heat.

2. Add the onion, garlic, turmeric, salt, and pepper and sauté until the vegetables are soft and translucent, 5 to 7 minutes.

3. Add the broth and squash and bring to a boil.

4. Reduce the heat to a simmer and cook until the squash has softened, about 5 minutes.

5. Add the shrimp and almond milk and cook until heated through, about 2 minutes.

6. Sprinkle with the almonds (if using), parsley, and lemon zest and serve.

TIPS: *If you're not a fan of shrimp, sole can be used instead. Cut the fish into 1-inch pieces, add the almond milk, and simmer until cooked through, about 5 minutes. This soup should be eaten within 48 hours of cooking.*

PER SERVING Calories: 275; Total Fat: 12g; Total Carbohydrates: 12g; Sugar: 3g; Fiber: 2g; Protein: 30g; Sodium: 1665mg

CLEAR CLAM CHOWDER

SERVES 4 / PREP TIME: 10 MINUTES / COOK TIME: 15 MINUTES

Most of us are used to cream- or tomato-based chowders. This chowder has all the flavor in the broth without any milk or acid from tomatoes. Since it uses canned, cooked clams, it's quick and easy to make.

2 tablespoons
  unsalted butter

2 medium carrots, cut into
  ½-inch pieces

2 celery stalks, thinly sliced

1 small red onion, cut into
  ¼-inch dice

2 garlic cloves, sliced

2 cups vegetable broth

1 (8-ounce) bottle clam juice

1 (10-ounce) can clams

½ teaspoon dried thyme

½ teaspoon salt

¼ teaspoon freshly ground
  black pepper

1. In a large pot, melt the butter over high heat.

2. Add the carrots, celery, onion, and garlic and sauté until slightly softened, 2 to 3 minutes.

3. Add the broth and clam juice and bring to a boil.

4. Reduce the heat to a simmer and cook until the carrots are soft, 3 to 5 minutes.

5. Stir in the clams and their juices, thyme, salt, and pepper, heat through for 2 to 3 minutes, and serve.

TIPS: *To make a creamy soup, add ½ cup full-fat coconut milk. Store this soup, covered, in the refrigerator for up to 48 hours, or freeze for several months.*

PER SERVING Calories: 156; Total Fat: 7g; Total Carbohydrates: 7g; Sugar: 3g; Fiber: 1g; Protein: 14g; Sodium: 981mg

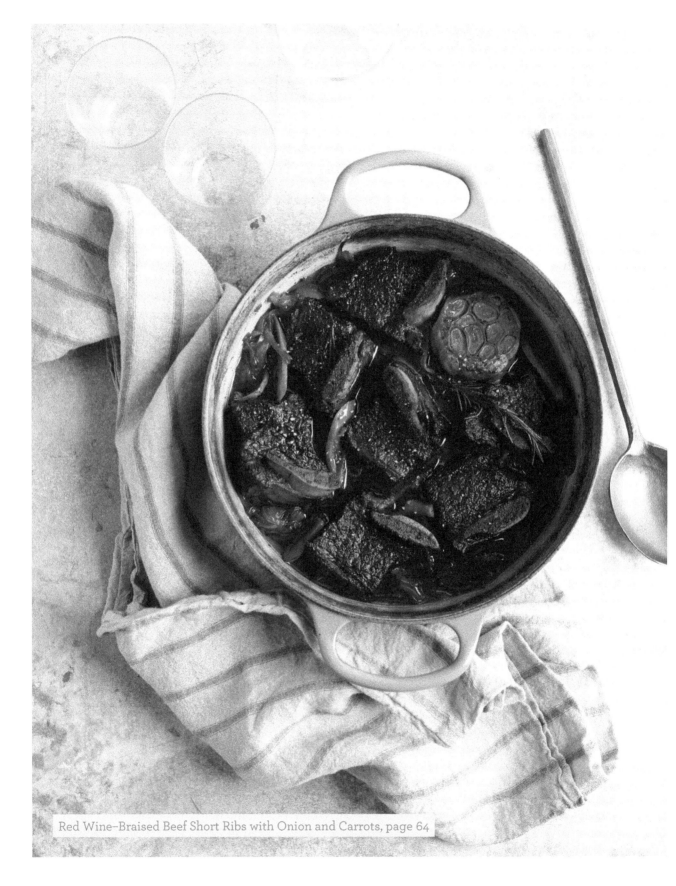

Red Wine–Braised Beef Short Ribs with Onion and Carrots, page 64

CHAPTER 5

Dutch Oven Dinners

The Dutch oven is one of the most important pieces of equipment in the kitchen. It can be used to sauté, simmer, fry, roast, and bake. Simmering food with the lid on concentrates the flavors and increases nutrition. Food cooked in a Dutch oven is typically hearty, and it's easy to make double batches and have leftovers throughout the week. Many of these recipes are braised, which means the food is cooked slowly with a small amount of liquid, resulting in proteins that are moist and tender. If you don't have a heavy enameled cast iron Dutch oven, a stainless steel one will work just as well.

WHITE BEAN CHILI

SERVES 4 / PREP TIME: 15 MINUTES / COOK TIME: 20 MINUTES

Using canned beans makes it easy to throw this chili together quickly. Cumin, the main spice in this chili, and oregano, decrease inflammation. This chili is great served over brown rice or quinoa and, if you'd like, garnished with sheep's milk feta or goat cheese.

¼ cup extra-virgin olive oil

2 small onions, cut into ¼-inch dice

2 celery stalks, thinly sliced

2 small carrots, peeled and thinly sliced

2 garlic cloves, minced

2 teaspoons ground cumin

1½ teaspoons dried oregano

1 teaspoon salt

¼ teaspoon freshly ground black pepper

3 cups vegetable broth

1 (15½-ounce) can white beans, drained and rinsed

¼ cup finely chopped fresh flat-leaf parsley

2 teaspoons grated or minced lemon zest

1. In a Dutch oven, heat the oil over high heat.

2. Add the onions, celery, carrots, and garlic and sauté until softened, 5 to 8 minutes.

3. Add the cumin, oregano, salt, and pepper and sauté to toast the spices, about 1 minute.

4. Add the broth and bring to a boil.

5. Reduce the heat to a simmer, add the beans, and cook, partially covered and stirring occasionally, for 5 minutes to develop the flavors.

6. Stir in the parsley and lemon zest and serve.

TIPS: *Ground turkey is a great addition to this recipe. Add to the recipe after Step 2, cook until browned, breaking it apart with a wooden spoon, for 5 to 7 minutes, then continue as written. Store, covered, in the refrigerator for up to 5 days, or freeze for several months.*

PER SERVING Calories: 300; Total Fat: 15g; Total Carbohydrates: 32g; Sugar: 4g; Fiber: 12g; Protein: 12g; Sodium: 1183mg

LAYERED GREEK-STYLE VEGETABLES

SERVES 4 / PREP TIME: 15 MINUTES / COOK TIME: 50 MINUTES

Vegetables are layered in a Dutch oven and baked, which makes this a great dish for entertaining, since there is no last-minute cooking. Serve ladled over a thick slice of gluten-free bread and drizzled with olive oil.

¼ cup extra-virgin olive oil

1 medium white onion, thinly sliced

2 large zucchini, thinly sliced

2 cups cauliflower florets

1 fennel bulb, trimmed and thinly sliced

2 garlic cloves, minced

1 teaspoon salt

¼ teaspoon freshly ground black pepper

2 cups vegetable broth

1 tablespoon chopped fresh dill

1½ teaspoons grated or minced lemon zest

½ cup crumbled sheep's or goat's milk feta cheese (optional)

1. Preheat the oven to 400°F.

2. Pour the oil into a Dutch oven. Arrange the onion in a single layer, and top, in layers, with the zucchini, cauliflower, fennel, garlic, salt, and pepper.

3. Pour the broth over the vegetables and sprinkle with the dill and lemon zest.

4. Cover the pot with the lid, transfer to the oven, and roast until the vegetables are tender, 30 to 40 minutes. Remove from the oven and let rest for about 10 minutes.

5. Sprinkle with the feta (if using) and serve.

TIPS: *You can easily add protein to this dish by adding drained cooked beans or cooked chicken sausage (without added sugars). Store, covered, in the refrigerator for up to 5 days, or freeze for several months.*

PER SERVING Calories: 200; Total Fat: 14g; Total Carbohydrates: 17g; Sugar: 6g; Fiber: 6g; Protein: 7g; Sodium: 1028mg

BAKED ZUCCHINI AND MUSHROOM RISOTTO

SERVES 4 / PREP TIME: 10 MINUTES / COOK TIME: 55 MINUTES

Classic risotto requires the cook to spend at least 45 minutes over the stove. In this recipe, the risotto is started on top of the stove and finished in the oven, shortening the time spent stirring to about 10 minutes. This is a family favorite, so you may want to make a double batch.

4 tablespoons (½ stick) unsalted butter

2 leeks, white parts only, thinly sliced

2 medium zucchini, thinly sliced

1 cup thinly sliced mushrooms

1 cup Arborio rice

½ cup white wine

2¼ cups vegetable broth

1 teaspoon salt

¼ teaspoon freshly ground black pepper

¼ teaspoon ground nutmeg

½ cup grated hard sheep's milk cheese, such as pecorino

1 tablespoon finely chopped fresh chives

1. Preheat the oven to 400°F.

2. In a Dutch oven, melt the butter over high heat.

3. Add the leeks and sauté until they begin to brown, for about 5 minutes.

4. Add the zucchini and mushrooms and sauté until softened and some of the liquid has evaporated, about 5 minutes.

5. Add the rice and cook until lightly browned, stirring, 3 to 4 minutes.

6. Add the wine, bring to a simmer, and cook until it evaporates, stirring, 3 to 4 minutes. Add the broth, salt, pepper, and nutmeg and bring to a boil.

7. Cover the pot, transfer to the oven, and bake until the rice is tender, 20 to 30 minutes. Remove from the oven, and let rest, covered, for 5 minutes to let the rice continue to cook.

8. Sprinkle with the cheese and chives and serve.

PER SERVING Calories: 417; Total Fat: 17g; Total Carbohydrates: 49g; Sugar: 4g; Fiber: 3g; Protein: 13g; Sodium: 1397mg

BUTTERNUT SQUASH AND QUINOA CHIPOTLE CHILI

SERVES 4 / PREP TIME: 10 MINUTES / COOK TIME: 50 MINUTES

Squash, quinoa, chipotle, and black beans comprise this chili. There are many types of salsas available in the markets; we like mango or pineapple salsa with this recipe.

3 tablespoons extra-virgin olive oil or coconut oil

1 medium red onion, cut into ¼-inch dice

1 garlic clove, minced

2 teaspoons chipotle chile powder

1 teaspoon ground cumin

1 teaspoon salt

½ teaspoon turmeric

¼ teaspoon freshly ground black pepper

2 cups peeled butternut squash cut into ½-inch dice

1 (15-ounce) can black beans, drained and rinsed

1 cup quinoa

2 scallions, both white and green parts, finely chopped

¼ cup finely chopped fresh cilantro

1. In a Dutch oven, heat the oil over high heat.

2. Add the onion and garlic and sauté until softened, 5 to 7 minutes.

3. Add the chile powder, cumin, salt, turmeric, and pepper and sauté to toast the spices, 1 to 2 minutes.

4. Add the squash, 2½ cups of water, beans, and quinoa and stir to mix well. Bring to a boil.

5. Reduce the heat to a simmer, partially cover, and cook until the squash and quinoa are tender, 20 to 30 minutes. Remove from the heat and let rest, covered, for 10 minutes.

6. Sprinkle with the scallions and cilantro and serve.

TIPS: *Brown rice can be substituted for the quinoa. If using brown rice, increase the cooking time by 10 minutes. Store, covered, in the refrigerator for up to 5 days, or freeze for several months.*

PER SERVING Calories: 385; Total Fat: 14g; Total Carbohydrates: 55g; Sugar: 3g; Fiber: 11g; Protein: 13g; Sodium: 609mg

MUSHROOM, KALE, AND SWEET POTATO BROWN RICE

SERVES 4 / PREP TIME: 10 MINUTES / COOK TIME: 50 MINUTES

The long cook time for this recipe is because of the brown rice. Feel free to substitute 3 cups cooked brown rice instead. If using cooked rice, this dish is ready to go in 10 minutes.

¼ cup extra-virgin olive oil

4 cups coarsely chopped kale leaves

2 leeks, white parts only, thinly sliced

1 cup sliced mushrooms

2 garlic cloves, minced

2 cups peeled sweet potatoes cut into ½-inch dice

1 cup brown rice

2 cups vegetable broth

1 teaspoon salt

¼ teaspoon freshly ground black pepper

¼ cup freshly squeezed lemon juice

2 tablespoons finely chopped fresh flat-leaf parsley

1. In a Dutch oven, heat the oil over high heat.

2. Add the kale, leeks, mushrooms, and garlic and sauté until soft, about 5 minutes.

3. Add the sweet potatoes and rice and sauté for about 3 minutes.

4. Add the broth, salt, and pepper and bring to a boil.

5. Reduce the heat to a simmer and cook, partially covered, until the rice is tender, 30 to 40 minutes.

6. Stir in the lemon juice and parsley and serve.

TIPS: *Feel free to substitute any green of choice for the kale. Swiss chard, mustard greens, or spinach all work well. Store, covered, in the refrigerator for up to 5 days, or freeze for several months.*

PER SERVING Calories: 425; Total Fat: 15g; Total Carbohydrates: 65g; Sugar: 6g; Fiber: 6g; Protein: 11g; Sodium: 1045mg

COCONUT CURRY CAULIFLOWER WITH CHICKPEAS

SERVES 4 / PREP TIME: 10 MINUTES / COOK TIME: 20 MINUTES

This is a light curry brightened by ginger and lemon. For best flavor, add the lemon zest right before serving.

¼ cup extra-virgin olive oil or coconut oil

1 medium onion, cut into ¼-inch dice

1 garlic clove, minced

1 (1-inch) piece fresh ginger, peeled and minced

2 medium carrots, peeled and thinly sliced

3 cups cauliflower florets

1 cup full-fat coconut milk

1 cup vegetable broth or water

2 teaspoons curry powder

1 teaspoon salt

1 (15-ounce) can chickpeas, drained and rinsed

2 scallions, both white and green parts, thinly sliced

2 tablespoons finely chopped fresh cilantro

2 teaspoons grated or minced lemon zest

1. In a Dutch oven, heat the oil over high heat.

2. Add the onion, garlic, and ginger and sauté to perfume the oil, about 3 minutes.

3. Add the carrots and sauté until softened, about 1 minute.

4. Add the cauliflower, coconut milk, broth, curry powder, and salt and bring to a boil.

5. Reduce the heat to a simmer and cook until the cauliflower is tender, 5 to 8 minutes.

6. Add the chickpeas and heat through, about 3 minutes.

7. Add the scallions, cilantro, and lemon zest, mix well, and serve.

TIPS: *This is great served over brown rice or quinoa. Store, covered, in the refrigerator for up to 5 days, or freeze for several months.*

PER SERVING Calories: 406; Total Fat: 29g; Total Carbohydrates: 32g; Sugar: 10g; Fiber: 10g; Protein: 10g; Sodium: 832mg

SPINACH AND FETA WITH BROWN RICE

SERVES 4 / PREP TIME: 10 MINUTES / COOK TIME: 50 MINUTES

This is a classic Greek dish containing rice and spinach. It's typically made with white rice, but brown rice provides better nutrition and adds a nuttiness to the dish.

4 tablespoons (½ stick) unsalted butter

4 scallions, both white and green parts, thinly sliced

1 garlic clove, thinly sliced

1 cup brown rice

2 cups vegetable broth

1 (10-ounce) package frozen chopped spinach, thawed and drained

1 teaspoon salt

¼ teaspoon freshly ground black pepper

½ cup crumbled sheep's milk feta cheese

1 tablespoon finely chopped fresh dill

1 tablespoon extra-virgin olive oil

1½ teaspoons grated or minced lemon zest

1. Preheat the oven to 400°F.

2. In a Dutch oven, melt the butter over high heat.

3. Add the scallions and garlic and sauté until softened, 1 to 2 minutes.

4. Add the rice and stir to coat the rice with the butter for about 1 minute.

5. Add the broth, spinach, salt, and pepper and bring to a boil.

6. Reduce the heat to a simmer, cover the pot, and transfer to the oven. Bake until the rice is tender, 30 to 40 minutes. Remove from the oven and let rest, covered, for 5 minutes.

7. Add the cheese, dill, oil, and lemon zest, mix to combine, and serve.

TIPS: *This dish can be eaten as an entrée or side dish. You can add 1 (15-ounce) can drained chickpeas to increase the protein. Store, covered, in the refrigerator for up to 5 days, or freeze for several months.*

PER SERVING Calories: 388; Total Fat: 21g; Total Carbohydrates: 42g; Sugar: 1g; Fiber: 4g; Protein: 11g; Sodium: 1242mg

CHINESE CHICKEN CASSEROLE WITH BROWN RICE

SERVES 4 / PREP TIME: 10 MINUTES / COOK TIME: 55 MINUTES

Ginger, garlic, and soy sauce are all the classic flavors of Asian cooking that perfume this dish.

¼ cup extra-virgin olive oil or coconut oil

2 garlic cloves, minced

1 (1-inch) piece fresh ginger, peeled and minced

1 pound boneless, skinless chicken breasts, cut into 1-inch pieces

2 cups chicken broth

2 cups broccoli florets

1 cup brown rice

1 teaspoon salt

¼ cup finely chopped fresh cilantro

2 scallions, both white and green parts, finely chopped

1 tablespoon gluten-free tamari or soy sauce

1 teaspoon sesame oil

¼ cup coarsely chopped cashews

1. In a Dutch oven, heat the olive oil over high heat.

2. Add the garlic and ginger and sauté until softened, about 1 minute.

3. Add the chicken and cook until lightly browned, about 5 minutes.

4. Add the broth, broccoli, rice, and salt and bring to a boil.

5. Reduce the heat to a simmer and cook, partially covered, until the rice is tender, 30 to 40 minutes. Remove from the heat and let rest, covered, for 5 minutes.

6. Remove the lid from the pot and add the cilantro, scallions, tamari, and sesame oil and mix well.

7. Sprinkle with the cashews and serve.

TIPS: *Store, covered, in the refrigerator for up to 5 days, or freeze for several months without the cashews. Add the cashews right before serving, or they will get soggy.*

PER SERVING Calories: 349; Total Fat: 23g; Total Carbohydrates: 8g; Sugar: 2g; Fiber: 2g; Protein: 29g; Sodium: 1039mg

GARLIC-ROASTED CHICKEN WITH CELERY

SERVES 4 / PREP TIME: 10 MINUTES / COOK TIME: 1¼ HOURS

This is a classic French preparation for roast chicken. Cooking it in a Dutch oven keeps the chicken very moist.

1 (3½- to 4-pound) chicken, patted dry with paper towels

1 teaspoon salt

4 tablespoons (½ stick) unsalted butter

3 celery stalks, thinly sliced

2 shallots, thinly sliced

1 carrot, peeled and thinly sliced

4 garlic cloves, peeled

½ cup white wine

1. Preheat the oven to 400°F.

2. Season the chicken with the salt.

3. In a Dutch oven, melt the butter over high heat.

4. Place the chicken, breast-side down, in the pot, and brown the breast meat for 3 to 4 minutes. Remove from the pot and set aside.

5. Add the celery, shallots, carrot, and garlic and sauté until softened, about 5 minutes.

6. Place the chicken, breast-side up, on top of the vegetables, and add 1 cup of water and the wine.

7. Cover the pot, transfer to the oven, and roast until the juices at the thigh are no longer pink, about 1 hour. Remove from the oven, and let rest for about 5 minutes before cutting into serving pieces.

8. Serve the chicken with the roasting vegetables and juices.

TIPS: *Leftover chicken can be used in many other recipes in this book. Store, covered, in the refrigerator for up to 5 days.*

PER SERVING Calories: 527; Total Fat: 35g; Total Carbohydrates: 7g; Sugar: 1g; Fiber: 1g; Protein: 39g; Sodium: 1085mg

CHICKEN AND APPLES OVER BRAISED RED CABBAGE

SERVES 4 / PREP TIME: 10 MINUTES / COOK TIME: 30 MINUTES

This is a satisfying dish for a fall or winter supper. Serve with brown rice or roasted sweet potatoes.

4 tablespoons (½ stick) unsalted butter

2 Granny Smith apples, cored, peeled, and cut into ½-inch pieces

1 large red onion, thinly sliced

2 celery stalks, thinly sliced

3 cups shredded red cabbage

1 tablespoon apple cider vinegar

1 cinnamon stick

1 teaspoon salt

½ teaspoon ground ginger

1 pound boneless, skinless chicken breasts, cut into 1-inch dice

2 teaspoons finely chopped fresh tarragon

1. Preheat the oven to 400°F.

2. In a Dutch oven, melt the butter over high heat.

3. Add the apples, onion, and celery and sauté until softened, about 5 minutes.

4. Add the cabbage, vinegar, cinnamon stick, salt, and ginger and cook until the cabbage wilts, about 3 minutes.

5. Place the chicken on top of the cabbage. Cover, transfer to the oven, and roast until the chicken is cooked through, about 15 minutes. Remove from the oven and let rest for about 5 minutes.

6. Sprinkle with the tarragon and serve.

TIPS: *If you have more time to cook, make this dish with chicken thighs with bones and skin. The bones and skin add lots of flavor to the dish but will extend the time in the oven to 45 minutes. Store, covered, in the refrigerator for up to 5 days.*

PER SERVING Calories: 319; Total Fat: 15g; Total Carbohydrates: 23g; Sugar: 15g; Fiber: 5g; Protein: 25g; Sodium: 739mg

TURKEY CUMIN BAKE

SERVES 4 / PREP TIME: 10 MINUTES / COOK TIME: 35 MINUTES

Cumin-scented roasted sweet potatoes, ground turkey, and white beans comprise this hearty dish. Place the goat cheese on top of the dish while hot from the oven so that it melts and becomes creamy.

¼ cup extra-virgin olive oil or coconut oil

1 pound ground turkey

2 cups peeled sweet potatoes cut into ½-inch dice

1 small red onion, cut into ¼-inch dice

1½ teaspoons dried oregano

1 teaspoon ground cumin

2 cups chicken broth

1 (15½-ounce) can white beans, drained and rinsed

6 ounces goat cheese, crumbled

1. Preheat the oven to 400°F.

2. In a Dutch oven, heat the oil over high heat.

3. Add the ground turkey and brown, breaking it up with a wooden spoon for 5 to 7 minutes.

4. Add the sweet potatoes, onion, oregano, and cumin and mix well.

5. Transfer the pot to the oven, and roast until the sweet potatoes are tender and lightly browned, 10 to 15 minutes.

6. Add the broth, stir in the beans, and return the pot to the oven to warm through for 2 to 4 minutes. Remove from the oven, and let rest, covered, for 5 minutes.

7. Sprinkle with the goat cheese on top, cover for 1 to 2 minutes to let it soften, and serve.

TIPS: *This dish can be made with butternut squash instead of sweet potatoes, and to keep it vegan you can omit the goat cheese. Store, covered, in the refrigerator for up to 5 days, or freeze for several months.*

PER SERVING Calories: 580; Total Fat: 31g; Total Carbohydrates: 34g; Sugar: 4g; Fiber: 10g; Protein: 34g; Sodium: 684mg

CHOCOLATE STEAK CHILI

SERVES 4 / PREP TIME: 15 MINUTES / COOK TIME: 30 MINUTES

Both the chocolate and cinnamon in this recipe are high in antioxidants and taste delicious. The sweetness of the winter squash complements the spice. If possible, it's best to buy organic, pastured beef.

¼ cup extra-virgin olive oil or coconut oil

1 pound boneless steak, cut into 1-inch pieces

1 large onion, thinly sliced

1 garlic clove, thinly sliced

1 tablespoon unsweetened cocoa powder

1 teaspoon chipotle chile powder

1 teaspoon salt

¼ teaspoon ground cinnamon

1 (15-ounce) can black beans, drained and rinsed

1 cup pumpkin or butternut squash purée

1 tablespoon apple cider vinegar

1. In a Dutch oven, heat the oil over high heat.

2. Add the steak and brown on all sides, about 5 minutes total. Remove from the pot and set aside.

3. Add the onion and garlic and sauté until softened, about 5 minutes.

4. Add the cocoa powder, chile powder, salt, and cinnamon and sauté to toast the spices for about 1 minute.

5. Return the steak to the pot and add the beans, pumpkin purée, 1 cup of water, and vinegar and bring to a simmer. Cook until the steak is tender, about 10 minutes. Remove from the heat, let rest for 5 minutes, and serve.

TIPS: *This dish is better eaten a day after it's made, so it's perfect as a make-ahead dish. Store, covered, in the refrigerator for up to 5 days, or freeze for several months.*

PER SERVING Calories: 387; Total Fat: 19g; Total Carbohydrates: 25g; Sugar: 4g; Fiber: 9g; Protein: 32g; Sodium: 661mg

RED WINE–BRAISED BEEF SHORT RIBS WITH ONION AND CARROTS

SERVES 4 / PREP TIME: 10 MINUTES / COOK TIME: 2¼ HOURS

Some things are worth waiting for, and short ribs are one of those things. They cook low and slow for about 2 hours, which is why we suggest making them on a weekend for a perfect reheat meal during the week. You can add any vegetables you like, and it's a good way to clean out the refrigerator.

4 tablespoons (½ stick) unsalted butter

2 pounds beef short ribs

1 teaspoon salt

¼ teaspoon freshly ground black pepper

2 cups chicken broth or water

1 cup red wine

1 medium onion, thinly sliced

2 medium carrots, peeled and thinly sliced

1 garlic head, halved horizontally

1 sprig fresh rosemary

1. Preheat the oven to 350°F.

2. In a Dutch oven, melt the butter over high heat.

3. Season the short ribs with the salt and pepper. Add to the pot, and brown on all sides, 5 to 8 minutes total.

4. Add the broth, wine, onion, carrots, garlic, and rosemary and bring to a boil.

5. Cover the pot, transfer to the oven, and roast until the short ribs are tender, 1½ to 2 hours. Remove from the oven, let rest for 5 minutes, and serve.

TIPS: *Serve with brown rice or mashed cauliflower. Store, covered, in the refrigerator for up to 5 days, or freeze for several months.*

PER SERVING Calories: 1085; Total Fat: 94g; Total Carbohydrates: 10g; Sugar: 4g; Fiber: 2g; Protein: 36g; Sodium: 1181mg

BAKED COD WITH LEMON AND SCALLIONS

SERVES 4 / PREP TIME: 15 MINUTES / COOK TIME: 35 MINUTES

Any firm-fleshed fish can be used in the recipe, including salmon, tuna, or swordfish.

2 tablespoons extra-virgin olive oil

1 lemon, thinly sliced

2 small carrots, peeled and thinly sliced

2 scallions, both white and green parts, cut into ½-inch pieces

1 garlic clove, sliced

1 pound skinless cod fillets

½ cup white wine

2 fresh thyme sprigs

1 teaspoon salt

¼ teaspoon freshly ground black pepper

1. Preheat the oven to 375°F. Coat the bottom of a Dutch oven with the oil.

2. Arrange the lemon slices on the bottom.

3. Add the carrots, scallions, and garlic.

4. Transfer the pot to the oven and bake until the carrots are soft, 5 to 10 minutes.

5. Place the cod on top of the vegetables and add the wine, thyme, salt, and pepper.

6. Cover the pot, return to the oven, and bake until the cod is just cooked through, 15 to 20 minutes. Remove from the oven. Let rest, covered, for 5 minutes and serve.

TIPS: *Leftovers of this dish can easily be made into a salad the next day by serving over a bed of greens and drizzling with olive oil and lemon juice. Store, covered, in the refrigerator for up to 48 hours. This dish does not freeze well.*

PER SERVING Calories: 193; Total Fat: 8g; Total Carbohydrates: 6g; Sugar: 2g; Fiber: 1g; Protein: 21g; Sodium: 682mg

BAKED MUSSELS AND LEEKS WITH SAFFRON

SERVES 4 / PREP TIME: 15 MINUTES / COOK TIME: 15 MINUTES

Fresh mussels are sold at markets that pride themselves on having a good seafood counter. This dish can be made with uncooked shrimp or clams. Serve with a leafy green salad and a gluten-free baguette or country loaf.

½ cup extra-virgin olive oil

2 leeks, white parts only, thinly sliced

2 celery stalks, thinly sliced

1 large carrot, peeled and thinly sliced

2 garlic cloves, minced

4 pounds mussels, rinsed and beards removed (just pull them off)

1 cup white wine

½ teaspoon salt

¼ teaspoon saffron threads

⅛ teaspoon red pepper flakes (optional)

2 tablespoons chopped fresh dill

Lemon wedges, for serving

1. In a large Dutch oven, heat the oil over high heat.

2. Add the leeks, celery, carrot, and garlic, and sauté until the onion is soft and translucent, about 5 minutes.

3. Add the mussels, wine, salt, saffron, and red pepper flakes (if using), cover, and bring to a boil.

4. Reduce the heat to medium, and cook, shaking the pot occasionally, until all the mussels have opened, 5 to 8 minutes.

5. Discard any unopened mussels, sprinkle with the dill, and serve with lemon wedges.

TIPS: *Some markets sell frozen cooked mussels. If making this dish with them, add the wine in Step 3, bring to a simmer, and add the defrosted mussels and heat through for about 5 minutes. Garnish with the dill and lemon wedges. This dish should be eaten shortly after being made.*

PER SERVING Calories: 388; Total Fat: 15g; Total Carbohydrates: 12g; Sugar: 3g; Fiber: 1g; Protein: 15g; Sodium: 642mg

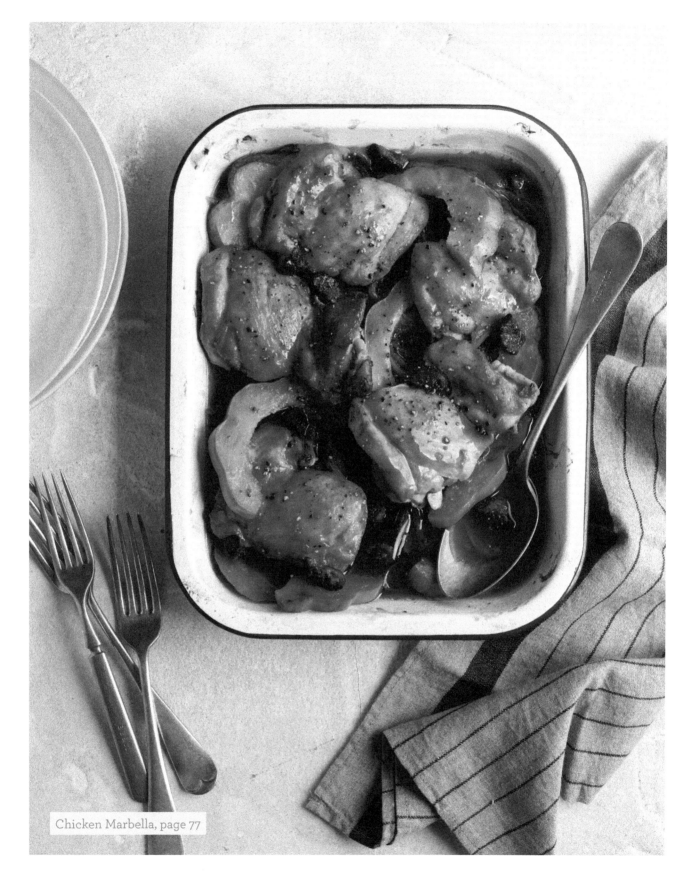

Chicken Marbella, page 77

CHAPTER 6

Hearty Casseroles

Casseroles are the workhorse of the kitchen. They are easy-to-create meals that can be made ahead of time and reheated when necessary, or covered and whisked off for a potluck, served piping hot for dinner. These recipes are designed to be crowd-pleasers, and even though most of the recipes are for an 8-by-8-inch dish, to serve four, they can all easily be doubled and made in a 9-by-13-inch dish to serve eight. When packing up leftovers, store in individual servings to make them easier to take to work for lunch.

SUMMER VEGETABLE FRITTATA

SERVES 4 / PREP TIME: 10 MINUTES / COOK TIME: 50 MINUTES

A classic frittata is made in a skillet and needs to be flipped halfway through, which can be challenging. This frittata is made entirely in the oven. The vegetables are first roasted in the pan, the eggs poured over, and the pan returned to the oven to cook through.

2 tablespoons extra-virgin olive oil

1 small red onion, thinly sliced

1 small zucchini, thinly sliced

1 (5-ounce) can artichoke hearts, drained and quartered

1 cup frozen corn, thawed

½ cup crumbled sheep's milk feta cheese

1 teaspoon dried oregano

½ teaspoon salt

10 large eggs, beaten

1. Preheat the oven to 375°F. Coat the bottom of an 8-by-8-inch casserole dish with the oil.

2. Arrange the onion and zucchini in an even layer in the dish.

3. Transfer the dish to the oven. Roast until the vegetables begin to caramelize, 5 to 7 minutes.

4. Add the artichoke hearts, corn, cheese, oregano, and salt.

5. Gently pour the eggs on top.

6. Return the dish to the oven. Bake until the eggs are firm but still jiggle a little when the dish is shaken, 25 to 35 minutes. Remove from the oven, let rest for 10 minutes, and serve.

TIPS: *You can use any vegetables you'd like in this recipe, and change it up seasonally. Try mushrooms and winter squash in the winter or asparagus and peas in the spring. Store, covered, in the refrigerator for up to 5 days. This will not freeze well.*

PER SERVING Calories: 341; Total Fat: 24g; Total Carbohydrates: 15g; Sugar: 4g; Fiber: 4g; Protein: 21g; Sodium: 643mg

SWEET POTATO–BROCCOLI GRATIN

SERVES 4 / PREP TIME: 15 MINUTES / COOK TIME: 25 MINUTES

This creamy dish can be either a side dish or an entrée. To add protein, choose beans, tofu, or salmon.

2 tablespoons coconut oil

2 cups peeled sweet potatoes cut into ½-inch dice

1 medium red onion, thinly sliced

2 cups broccoli florets

2 cups coconut milk or almond milk

1 teaspoon salt

⅛ teaspoon freshly ground black pepper

4 ounces goat cheese cheese, crumbled

1. Preheat the oven to 375°F. Coat the bottom of an 8-by-8-inch casserole dish with the oil.

2. Add the sweet potatoes and onion.

3. Transfer the dish to the oven, and roast until the sweet potatoes are tender, about 10 minutes.

4. Add the broccoli, coconut milk, salt, and pepper. Stir to mix.

5. Return the dish to the oven, and bake until bubbly and lightly browned, about 15 minutes.

6. Sprinkle the cheese on top and serve.

TIPS: *This can be made with winter squash instead of sweet potatoes, and if you have a nut allergy, substitute vegetable broth for the coconut milk or almond milk. Store, covered, in the refrigerator for up to 5 days, or freeze for several months.*

PER SERVING Calories: 494; Total Fat: 42g; Total Carbohydrates: 29g; Sugar: 9g; Fiber: 6g; Protein: 11g; Sodium: 756mg

ZUCCHINI AND QUINOA BAKE WITH GOAT CHEESE

SERVES 4 / PREP TIME: 10 MINUTES / COOK TIME: 35 MINUTES

Zucchini, quinoa, white beans, walnuts, and goat cheese comprise this delicious high-fiber, high-protein dinner. This recipe will be so popular with your family, you'll want to make a double batch.

2 tablespoons extra-virgin olive oil

½ cup quinoa

2 small zucchini, thinly sliced

1 cup canned white beans, drained and rinsed

2 scallions, both white and green parts, thinly sliced

1 garlic clove, minced

1 cup vegetable broth

1 teaspoon salt

½ teaspoon dried thyme

2 ounces goat cheese cheese, crumbled

¼ cup coarsely chopped walnuts (optional)

1. Preheat the oven to 375°F. Coat the bottom of an 8-by-8-inch casserole dish with the oil.

2. Spread the quinoa evenly in the dish.

3. Place the zucchini, beans, scallions, and garlic on top of the quinoa.

4. Carefully pour the broth over the vegetables and season with the salt and thyme.

5. Cover the dish, transfer to the oven, and bake until the quinoa is tender, about 25 minutes. Remove from the oven and let rest, covered, for 5 to 10 minutes.

6. Sprinkle with the cheese and walnuts (if using) and serve.

TIPS: *If using cooked quinoa, use 2 cups, and reduce the cooking time to 15 minutes. If vegan, omit the goat cheese. Store, covered, in the refrigerator for up to 5 days, or freeze for several months.*

PER SERVING Calories: 264; Total Fat: 12g; Total Carbohydrates: 31g; Sugar: 2g; Fiber: 6g; Protein: 13g; Sodium: 858mg

QUINOA AND CARROT CASSEROLE WITH TURMERIC AND CUMIN

SERVES 4 / PREP TIME: 10 MINUTES / COOK TIME: 45 MINUTES

Turmeric and cumin are anti-inflammatory stars and season the quinoa, which makes up the base of this casserole. The carrots and parsnip are roasted in the casserole first, adding their sweetness to the dish.

⅓ cup extra-virgin olive oil

2 medium carrots, cut into ¼-inch-thick slices

1 large parsnip, cut into ¼-inch-thick slices

2 tablespoons balsamic vinegar

1 teaspoon salt

1 teaspoon turmeric

½ teaspoon ground cumin

¼ teaspoon freshly ground black pepper

1 cup quinoa

2 cups vegetable broth

2 scallions, both white and green parts, thinly sliced

1. Preheat the oven to 400°F.

2. In a 9-by-13-inch casserole dish, combine the oil, carrots, parsnip, vinegar, salt, turmeric, cumin, and pepper.

3. Transfer the dish to the oven and roast until the vegetables begin to brown and soften, about 10 minutes.

4. Evenly distribute the quinoa over the vegetables, add the broth, and sprinkle with the scallions.

5. Cover the dish, return to the oven, and roast until the quinoa is cooked through, about 30 minutes. Remove from the oven, and let rest, covered, for 5 minutes.

6. Fluff the quinoa with a fork and serve.

TIPS: *This is cooked in a 9-by-13-inch dish so that the quinoa cooks more quickly. Store, covered, in the refrigerator for up to 5 days, or freeze for several months.*

PER SERVING Calories: 364; Total Fat: 20g; Total Carbohydrates: 38g; Sugar: 4g; Fiber: 6g; Protein: 9g; Sodium: 992mg

BAKED CAULIFLOWER IN COCONUT MILK WITH CILANTRO

SERVES 4 / PREP TIME: 10 MINUTES / COOK TIME: 25 MINUTES

Coconut milk makes this gratin creamy, and the garlic, ginger, and turmeric enhance the delicate flavor of cauliflower. If you don't like coconut milk, substitute unsweetened almond milk. Many markets sell cauliflower florets in the produce department, which are perfect in this recipe.

¼ cup coconut oil or extra-virgin olive oil

3 cups cauliflower florets

2 cups full-fat coconut milk

1 garlic clove, thinly sliced

1 teaspoon salt

1 teaspoon turmeric

½ teaspoon ground ginger

¼ teaspoon freshly ground black pepper

2 scallions, both white and green parts, thinly sliced

1 tablespoon finely chopped fresh cilantro

1. Preheat the oven to 400°F. Coat the bottom of an 8-by-8-inch casserole dish with the oil.

2. Add the cauliflower, coconut milk, garlic, salt, turmeric, ginger, and pepper.

3. Cover the dish, transfer to the oven, and roast until the cauliflower is tender, about 15 minutes.

4. Uncover the dish, return to the oven, and roast until bubbly, 5 to 8 minutes.

5. Sprinkle with the scallions and cilantro and serve.

TIPS: *The cauliflower will cook faster when cut smaller. It's easy to add protein to make this a more complete meal: Tofu, beans, and chicken are all good options. Store, covered, in the refrigerator for up to 5 days, or freeze for several months.*

PER SERVING Calories: 419; Total Fat: 42g; Total Carbohydrates: 12g; Sugar: 6g; Fiber: 5g; Protein: 5g; Sodium: 624mg

BROWN RICE AND VEGETABLE CASSEROLE

SERVES 4 / PREP TIME: 10 MINUTES / COOK TIME: 1 HOUR

This dish is cooked in a larger 9-by-13-inch casserole so that the rice cooks faster; however, you can make this dish with cooked brown rice instead. If using cooked rice, use 3 cups of cooked rice instead of 1 cup of uncooked rice and only add ½ cup of vegetable broth.

¼ cup extra-virgin olive oil

1 small red onion, thinly sliced

1 small sweet potato, peeled and thinly sliced

1 cup broccoli florets

1 garlic clove, thinly sliced

1 teaspoon salt

1 teaspoon dried thyme

¼ teaspoon freshly ground black pepper

2 cups vegetable broth

1 cup medium-grain brown rice

¼ cup freshly squeezed lemon juice

1. Preheat the oven to 400°F. Coat the bottom of a 9-by-13-inch casserole dish with the oil.

2. Add the onion, sweet potato, broccoli, garlic, salt, thyme, and pepper and toss until well mixed.

3. Transfer the dish to the oven and roast until the vegetables have softened, about 10 minutes.

4. Add the broth and rice and stir to combine.

5. Cover the dish, return to the oven, and bake until the rice is tender, 30 to 40 minutes. Remove from the oven and let rest, covered, for 10 minutes.

6. Carefully uncover the dish, add the lemon juice, fluff the rice with a fork, and serve.

TIPS: *Use seasonal vegetables for this dish. The dish can be made more substantial with the addition of proteins like beans, tofu, or chicken. Store, covered, in the refrigerator for up to 5 days, or freeze for several months.*

PER SERVING Calories: 333; Total Fat:15g; Total Carbohydrates: 44g; Sugar: 3g; Fiber: 3g; Protein: 7g; Sodium: 983mg

GARLICKY CANNELLINI BEANS

SERVES 4 TO 6 / PREP TIME: 10 MINUTES / COOK TIME: 15 MINUTES

Swiss chard, cannellini beans, and garlic are the base for this dish. Using canned beans makes this quick to prepare. Serve hot, with olive oil for drizzling and gluten-free bread to sop up the juices.

1 large bunch Swiss chard, leaves only, cut into 2-inch strips

1 (15-ounce) can cannellini beans, drained and rinsed

1 cup vegetable broth

½ small onion, chopped

¼ cup extra-virgin olive oil

2 garlic cloves, thinly sliced

1 teaspoon grated or minced lemon zest

1 teaspoon salt

½ teaspoon dried rosemary

2 tablespoons freshly squeezed lemon juice

1. Preheat the oven to 400°F.

2. In an 8-by-8-inch casserole dish, combine the Swiss chard, beans, broth, onion, oil, garlic, lemon zest, salt, and rosemary and stir until well mixed.

3. Cover the dish, transfer to the oven, and bake until the chard has wilted and the beans are thoroughly heated, 10 to 15 minutes.

4. Stir in the lemon juice and serve.

TIPS: *Leftovers are great eaten as a salad. Store, covered, in the refrigerator for up to 5 days, or freeze for several months.*

PER SERVING Calories: 217; Total Fat: 14g; Total Carbohydrates: 18g; Sugar: 1g; Fiber: 6g; Protein: 8g; Sodium: 853mg

CHICKEN MARBELLA

SERVES 4 / PREP TIME: 15 MINUTES / COOK TIME: 55 MINUTES

Chicken Marbella is a classic that never disappoints. Traditionally it is made with whole pieces of chicken on the bone, but we used boneless chicken for a shorter cooking time.

2 tablespoons unsalted butter, at room temperature

1 acorn squash, seeded and thinly sliced

½ cup coarsely chopped prunes or dried figs

½ onion, thinly sliced

1 garlic clove, thinly sliced

2 pounds bone-in, skin-on chicken thighs

1 tablespoon honey

1 teaspoon salt

1 cup chicken broth

1. Preheat the oven to 375°F. Coat the bottom of an 8-by-8-inch casserole dish with the butter.

2. Evenly distribute the squash, prunes, onion, and garlic in the dish.

3. Place the chicken on top of the vegetables, drizzle with the honey, and season with the salt.

4. Add the broth, cover the dish, and transfer to the oven. Bake until the chicken is cooked through, 35 to 45 minutes. Remove from the oven. Let rest, covered, for 10 minutes and serve.

TIPS: *It's fine to substitute boneless chicken breast for the chicken thighs. If using chicken breast, the chicken may cook faster; check after 20 minutes. Store, covered, in the refrigerator for up to 5 days, or freeze for several months.*

PER SERVING Calories: 723; Total Fat: 49g; Total Carbohydrates: 33g; Sugar: 17g; Fiber: 4g; Protein: 41g; Sodium: 978mg

DAIRY, NUTS

CHICKEN FLORENTINE

SERVES 4 / PREP TIME: 10 MINUTES / COOK TIME: 35 MINUTES

This is a creamy chicken and spinach casserole, with coconut milk replacing the cream. Coconut milk has a high fat content, which makes it a good substitute for cream, but if you don't like the taste of coconut milk, feel free to use unsweetened almond milk instead.

2 tablespoons extra-virgin olive oil

3 cups baby spinach

½ cup thinly sliced mushrooms

2 scallions, both white and green parts, thinly sliced

2 pounds boneless, skinless chicken breasts

½ cup full-fat coconut milk

1 teaspoon salt

¼ teaspoon freshly ground black pepper

¼ cup grated sheep's milk pecorino cheese

1. Preheat the oven to 375°F. Coat the bottom of an 8-by-8-inch casserole dish with the oil.

2. Evenly distribute the spinach in the dish.

3. Scatter the mushrooms and scallions over the spinach.

4. Add the chicken, coconut milk, salt, and pepper.

5. Cover the dish, transfer to the oven, and bake until the chicken is cooked through, 20 to 25 minutes. Remove from the oven, and let rest, covered, for 10 minutes.

6. Sprinkle with the cheese and serve.

TIPS: *If you have nut sensitivities, use white wine instead of the coconut milk. Store, covered, in the refrigerator for up to 5 days, or freeze for several months.*

PER SERVING Calories: 418; Total Fat: 22g; Total Carbohydrates: 3g; Sugar: 1g; Fiber: 2g; Protein: 51g; Sodium: 860mg

CHICKEN, BROCCOLI, AND BROWN RICE BAKE

SERVES 4 / PREP TIME: 10 MINUTES / COOK TIME: 50 MINUTES

A twist on a classic chicken and rice, this version uses brown rice and adds broccoli.

2 tablespoons extra-virgin olive oil

½ cup brown rice

1 pound boneless, skinless chicken breasts, cut into 1-inch pieces

2 cups broccoli florets

2 scallions, both white and green parts, thinly sliced

1 cup chicken broth

1 teaspoon salt

¼ teaspoon freshly ground black pepper

1. Preheat the oven to 375°F. Coat the bottom of an 8-by-8-inch casserole dish with the oil.

2. Spread the rice evenly over the bottom of the dish.

3. Place the chicken, broccoli, and scallions on top of the rice.

4. Add the broth and season with the salt and pepper.

5. Cover the dish, transfer to the oven, and bake until the rice is tender and the chicken is cooked through, 30 to 40 minutes. Remove from the oven, let rest, covered, for 5 to 10 minutes and serve.

TIPS: *Simplify this casserole even more by using cooked brown rice and cooked chicken. Follow the directions as written but shorten the time in the oven to 15 to 20 minutes, or until the rice and chicken are heated through and the broccoli is tender. Store, covered, in the refrigerator for up to 5 days, or freeze for several months.*

PER SERVING Calories: 301; Total Fat: 11g; Total Carbohydrates: 22g; Sugar: 1g; Fiber: 2g; Protein: 28g; Sodium: 847mg

SALMON AND APRICOTS OVER BROWN RICE

SERVES 4 / PREP TIME: 10 MINUTES / COOK TIME: 30 MINUTES

This dish is best made with ripe fresh apricots, but since apricots have a short season, it's fine to use thawed frozen apricots instead. We like to serve this dish with a simple coleslaw.

2 tablespoons unsalted butter, at room temperature

1 leek, white part only, thinly sliced

½ cup brown rice

1 cup vegetable broth

1 pound skinless salmon fillets

4 apricots, halved and pitted

¼ cup white wine

1 teaspoon salt

¼ teaspoon freshly ground black pepper

¼ teaspoon dried thyme

1. Preheat the oven to 375°F. Coat the bottom of an 8-by-8-inch casserole dish with the butter.

2. Arrange the leek in an even layer in the dish, and evenly distribute the rice over the leeks.

3. Add the broth, cover the dish, and transfer to the oven. Partially bake the rice for about 10 minutes.

4. Add the salmon, apricots, and the wine and season with the salt, pepper, and thyme.

5. Cover the dish, return to the oven, and bake until the rice is tender and the salmon is cooked through, about 20 minutes.

TIPS: *If using cooked brown rice, you will need 2 cups for this recipe. You can use dried apricots; they will turn plump, but still have a firm texture. Store, covered, in the refrigerator, and eat within 48 hours.*

PER SERVING Calories: 390; Total Fat: 19g; Total Carbohydrates: 26g; Sugar: 4g; Fiber: 2g; Protein: 26g; Sodium: 885mg

LENTIL AND TUNA CASSEROLE WITH SPINACH AND GINGER

SERVES 4 / PREP TIME: 10 MINUTES / COOK TIME: 15 MINUTES

This dish uses canned tuna but can be made with canned salmon instead, if desired. The nuttiness of lentils works well with the tuna and ginger, and scallions brighten the dish. To make a more complete meal, serve with brown rice.

4 cups baby spinach

1 (15-ounce) can lentils, drained and rinsed

2 (5-ounce) cans water-packed tuna, drained

2 teaspoons minced peeled fresh ginger

½ teaspoon salt

¼ teaspoon freshly ground black pepper

2 teaspoons extra-virgin olive oil

2 tablespoons red-wine vinegar

2 scallions, both white and green parts, thinly sliced

1. Preheat the oven to 375°F.

2. In a 9-by-13-inch casserole dish, combine the spinach, lentils, tuna, ginger, salt, and pepper and mix well.

3. Drizzle with the oil and vinegar and sprinkle with the scallions.

4. Cover the dish, transfer to the oven, and bake until hot, 10 to 15 minutes. Remove from the oven and serve.

TIPS: *The easiest way to grate ginger is to use a Microplane. If you don't have one, use the finest holes on a cheese grater. Even though this recipe serves four, it's made in a 9-by-13-inch dish so that there's enough room to accommodate the spinach. Once cooked, the spinach will significantly decrease in size. Store, covered, in the refrigerator for up to 5 days. This dish doesn't freeze well.*

PER SERVING Calories: 213; Total Fat: 3g; Total Carbohydrates: 17g; Sugar: 2g; Fiber: 7g; Protein: 29g; Sodium: 359mg

BAKED SCAMPI CASSEROLE

SERVES 4 / PREP TIME: 10 MINUTES / COOK TIME: 15 MINUTES

Butter and garlic give this dish its signature flavor, and the asparagus adds nutrition and fiber.

2 tablespoons unsalted
butter, at room
temperature

1 pound peeled shrimp,
thawed if necessary

2 cups pencil-width
asparagus cut into
1-inch pieces

1 cup white wine

2 garlic cloves, minced

2 tablespoons finely
chopped fresh
flat-leaf parsley

1. Preheat the oven to 375°F. Coat the bottom of an 8-by-8-inch casserole dish with the butter.

2. Add the shrimp, asparagus, wine, and garlic.

3. Cover the dish, transfer to the oven, and bake until the shrimp are pink and the asparagus has softened, about 15 minutes. Remove from the oven and uncover carefully, as steam will escape.

4. Sprinkle with the parsley and serve.

TIPS: *Leftovers can be served on top of salad greens and eaten cold. Store, covered, in the refrigerator for up to 24 hours. This will not freeze well.*

PER SERVING Calories: 224; Total Fat: 7g; Total Carbohydrates: 5g; Sugar: 2g; Fiber: 2g; Protein: 26g; Sodium: 303mg

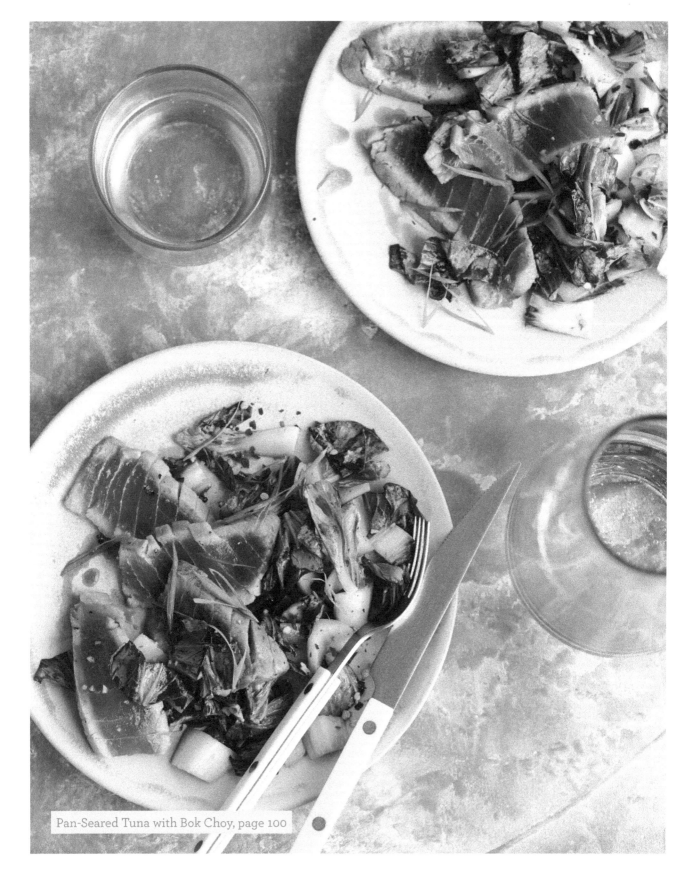

Pan-Seared Tuna with Bok Choy, page 100

CHAPTER 7

Skillful Skillets

The best skillet for these recipes is one that can go from the stove to the oven, since many proteins are seared in the skillet and finished in the oven (or toaster oven). For four servings, the skillet should be at least 12 inches in diameter. Skillet cooking is perfect for roasting and searing, since foods can be cooked over high heat. The beauty of cooking in a skillet is you can serve out of it as well, leaving only one pan to clean. The quick searing of vegetables keeps the nutrient levels high.

SPINACH AND MUSHROOMS WITH EGGS AND GOAT CHEESE

SERVES 4 / PREP TIME: 10 MINUTES / COOK TIME: 20 MINUTES

This can be served at breakfast as easily as dinner, or for a weekend brunch. For best nutrition look for organic, pastured eggs. Olives are a good addition.

2 tablespoons extra-virgin olive oil

1 cup thinly sliced mushrooms

2 scallions, both white and green parts, thinly sliced

4 cups baby spinach

1 teaspoon salt

¼ teaspoon red pepper flakes (optional)

4 large eggs

½ cup crumbled goat cheese cheese

2 teaspoons finely chopped fresh dill

1. Preheat the oven to 400°F.

2. In an oven-safe skillet, heat the oil over high heat. Add the mushrooms and scallions and sauté until the liquid from the mushrooms has evaporated, 3 to 5 minutes.

3. Add the spinach, salt, and red pepper flakes (if using) and cook until the spinach has wilted, about 2 minutes.

4. Use the back of a spoon to create four evenly distributed wells in the spinach.

5. Crack an egg into a small bowl and gently pour it into one of the wells. Repeat with the remaining eggs.

6. Transfer the skillet to the oven, and bake until the eggs are your desired firmness, 10 to 12 minutes for eggs that are still soft.

7. Sprinkle with the cheese and dill and serve.

TIPS: *Swiss chard is a good substitute for spinach in this dish. This should be eaten shortly after it's made.*

PER SERVING Calories: 184; Total Fat: 15g; Total Carbohydrates: 3g; Sugar: 1g; Fiber: 1g; Protein: 11g; Sodium: 730mg

QUINOA, ROOT VEGETABLES, AND CHICKPEAS

SERVES 4 / PREP TIME: 10 MINUTES / COOK TIME: 30 MINUTES

This whole meal is cooked on top of the stove. The vegetables are sautéed, then quinoa, broth, and chickpeas are all simmered until tender. The flat surface of a skillet speeds up cooking time, and the quinoa and chickpeas add protein and fiber.

2 tablespoons extra-virgin olive oil or coconut oil

½ red onion, thinly sliced

1 garlic clove, minced

1 large carrot, cut into ½-inch dice

1 parsnip, cut into ½-inch dice

1 large golden beet, peeled and cut into ½-inch dice

1 cup quinoa

1 teaspoon salt

¼ teaspoon freshly ground black pepper

2 cups vegetable broth

1 cup canned chickpeas, drained and rinsed

2 tablespoons finely chopped fresh mint

1. In a skillet, heat the oil over high heat.

2. Add the onion and garlic and sauté until softened, about 2 minutes.

3. Add the carrot, parsnip, beet, quinoa, salt, and pepper and stir until well combined.

4. Add the broth and chickpeas and bring to a boil.

5. Reduce the heat to a simmer and cook, stirring occasionally, until the quinoa is tender, about 20 minutes. Remove from the heat, cover, and let rest for 5 minutes.

6. Sprinkle with the mint and serve.

TIPS: *This can be made with cooked quinoa. If using cooked quinoa, use 3 cups, decrease the vegetable broth to ½ cup, and cook only until the vegetables are tender. Store, covered, in the refrigerator, for up to 5 days, or freeze for several months.*

PER SERVING Calories: 311; Total Fat: 11g; Total Carbohydrates: 43g; Sugar: 6g; Fiber: 7g; Protein: 11g; Sodium: 804mg

VEGAN

POLENTA AND MUSHROOMS

SERVES 4 / PREP TIME: 10 MINUTES / COOK TIME: 40 MINUTES

Look for organic polenta, since nonorganic has most likely been genetically modified. We like to change the vegetables depending on the season: using winter squash in the fall and winter, peas in the spring, and asparagus in the summer. Add beans, fish, or shrimp to this recipe to increase the protein.

2 tablespoons extra-virgin olive oil

1 shallot, thinly sliced

2 cups thinly sliced mushrooms

½ cup white wine

1 teaspoon salt

¼ teaspoon ground nutmeg

1 cup polenta or grits

2 cups vegetable broth

½ cup chopped scallions, both white and green parts

1. In a medium skillet, heat the oil over high heat.

2. Add the shallot and sauté until softened, about 1 minute.

3. Add the mushrooms, wine, salt, and nutmeg and cook until the wine has evaporated, 3 to 5 minutes.

4. Add the polenta and stir to evenly mix.

5. Stirring constantly, add the broth in a thin, steady stream, and bring to a boil.

6. Reduce the heat to a simmer, and cook, stirring frequently, until all the liquid has been absorbed and the polenta is tender, 15 to 20 minutes. Remove from the heat and let rest, covered, for 5 to 10 minutes.

7. Sprinkle with the scallions and serve.

TIPS: *Polenta, grits, or medium-grain cornmeal can all be used in this recipe. Store this dish, covered, in the refrigerator for up to 5 days, or freeze for several months.*

PER SERVING Calories: 256; Total Fat: 8g; Total Carbohydrates: 34g; Sugar: 2g; Fiber: 2g; Protein: 7g; Sodium: 970mg

SWISS CHARD AND ARBORIO RICE

SERVES 4 / PREP TIME: 10 MINUTES / COOK TIME: 45 MINUTES

Arborio is a thick short-grain rice. This recipe is vegan, but if you want a creamier rice, add ½ cup goat cheese right before serving.

¼ cup extra-virgin olive oil

½ onion, cut into ¼-inch dice

1 garlic clove, minced

3 cups stemmed Swiss chard leaves cut into 1-inch pieces

1 teaspoon salt

¼ teaspoon freshly ground black pepper

1 cup Arborio rice

2½ cups vegetable broth, divided

1 tablespoon finely chopped fresh flat-leaf parsley

1. In a medium skillet, heat the oil over high heat. Add the onion and garlic and sauté until softened, 1 to 2 minutes. Add the Swiss chard, salt, and pepper and cook until wilted, about 2 minutes.

2. Add the rice and stir until well mixed and coated with the oil, about 2 minutes.

3. Add 1 cup of broth and cook, stirring occasionally, until it has been absorbed, about 5 minutes.

4. Add another cup of broth and repeat the previous step.

5. Add the remaining ½ cup of broth and stir until absorbed and the rice is tender, 15 to 20 minutes.

6. Let the rice rest for 5 to 10 minutes, add the parsley, and serve.

TIPS: *Store, covered, in the refrigerator for up to 5 days, or freeze for several months. Arborio rice is typically sold in the rice or international food sections of the market, where you'll find both imported and domestically grown varieties. The domestic rice is less expensive and just as good.*

PER SERVING Calories: 316; Total Fat: 14g; Total Carbohydrates: 41g; Sugar: 1g; Fiber: 2g; Protein: 7g; Sodium: 1121mg

SKILLET GLUTEN-FREE PIZZA WITH FIGS, CARAMELIZED ONION, AND GOAT CHEESE

SERVES 4 / PREP TIME: 10 MINUTES / COOK TIME: 20 MINUTES

This skillet is super easy to make when using premade gluten-free pizza dough. In this recipe, we are using onion and figs, but asparagus or mushrooms are also good options.

2 tablespoons extra-virgin olive oil

1 small red onion, thinly sliced

1 garlic clove, minced

1 teaspoon salt

¼ teaspoon red pepper flakes (optional)

1 (10-inch) premade gluten-free pizza shell

4 large ripe figs, halved

½ cup crumbled goat cheese cheese

1 tablespoon balsamic vinegar

½ teaspoon dried rosemary

1. Preheat the oven to 400°F.

2. In a medium oven-safe skillet, heat the oil over high heat. Add the onion and garlic and sauté until the onion is golden, 5 to 8 minutes. Season with the salt and red pepper flakes (if using), remove from the skillet, and set aside.

3. Fit the pizza shell into the skillet (you don't have to clean it), and evenly distribute the onion and garlic, figs, and cheese over the shell. Drizzle with the vinegar and sprinkle with the rosemary.

4. Transfer the skillet to the oven and bake until the crust is lightly browned and the cheese is soft, about 10 minutes. Remove from the oven, cut into eight wedges, and serve.

TIPS: *Gluten-free pizza shells can be found in the freezer, bread, or flatbread aisles of the grocery store. This pizza should be eaten shortly after it's baked, but can be frozen unbaked for several weeks.*

PER SERVING Calories: 235; Total Fat: 12g; Total Carbohydrates: 30g; Sugar: 13g; Fiber: 3g; Protein: 5g; Sodium: 780mg

VEGAN

GINGER TOFU AND BOK CHOY SKILLET

SERVES 4 / PREP TIME: 10 MINUTES / COOK TIME: 15 MINUTES

Purchase firm tofu for this recipe, and look for organic tofu, since non-organic tofu has most likely been genetically modified. Brown rice is a great side dish for this recipe.

2 tablespoons sesame oil

1 garlic clove, minced

1 (1½-inch) piece
   fresh ginger, peeled
   and minced

3 cups bok choy cut into
   1-inch pieces

1 pound firm tofu, cut into
   1-inch dice

½ cup vegetable broth

1½ teaspoons gluten-free
   tamari or soy sauce

2 scallions, both white and
   green parts, thinly sliced

1 tablespoon finely
   chopped fresh cilantro

1. In a large skillet, heat the oil over high heat.

2. Add the garlic and ginger and stir-fry until softened, about 1 minute.

3. Add the bok choy, and stir-fry until wilted, 2 to 3 minutes.

4. Add the tofu, broth, and tamari and stir-fry until all the ingredients are evenly mixed and the tofu is heated through, 5 to 8 minutes.

5. Sprinkle with the scallions and cilantro and serve.

TIPS: *Tempeh can be substituted for the tofu, since many people find tempeh more digestible. Broccolini or spinach can be substituted for the bok choy. Store, covered, in the refrigerator for up to 5 days, or freeze for several months.*

PER SERVING Calories: 156; Total Fat: 12g; Total Carbohydrates: 4g; Sugar: 2g; Fiber: 2g; Protein: 11g; Sodium: 257mg

CHICKEN, KALE, AND WALNUT SKILLET

SERVES 4 / PREP TIME: 10 MINUTES / COOK TIME: 35 MINUTES

This hearty skillet is made creamy with coconut milk, but feel free to substitute unsweetened almond milk instead, or if you are sensitive to nuts, use chicken broth. The nuttiness of brown rice makes it the perfect side dish.

2 tablespoons unsalted butter

4 boneless, skinless chicken thighs

1 teaspoon salt

¼ teaspoon freshly ground black pepper

½ red onion, cut into ¼-inch dice

3 cups stemmed kale leaves cut into 1-inch strips

1 cup full-fat coconut milk

½ cup coarsely chopped walnuts

1. Preheat the oven to 400°F.

2. In an oven-safe skillet, melt the butter over high heat.

3. Add the chicken and brown on both sides, 2 to 3 minutes per side. Season with the salt and pepper, remove from the skillet, and set aside.

4. Add the onion and kale and sauté until the kale has wilted, about 1 minute.

5. Return the chicken to the skillet, add the coconut milk, and transfer to the oven. Bake until the chicken is cooked through, about 20 minutes. Remove from the oven and let rest, covered, for 5 minutes.

6. Sprinkle with the walnuts and serve.

TIPS: *This recipe can be made with boneless, skinless chicken breast instead of thighs. Store, covered, in the refrigerator for up to 5 days, or freeze for several months.*

PER SERVING Calories: 403; Total Fat: 30g; Total Carbohydrates: 11g; Sugar: 3g; Fiber: 3g; Protein: 26g; Sodium: 754mg

CHICKEN AND SPRING VEGETABLES WITH BROWN RICE SKILLET

SERVES 4 / PREP TIME: 10 MINUTES / COOK TIME: 40 MINUTES

This skillet is a twist on a classic chicken and rice dish. The recipe is seasoned with the Mediterranean flavors of oregano and mint, but you can substitute those with jalapeños and cilantro, or ginger and soy to stave off dinner boredom.

2 tablespoons unsalted butter

1 pound boneless, skinless chicken breasts, cut into 1-inch pieces

1 pound asparagus, trimmed of woody ends and cut into 1-inch pieces

1 cup frozen green peas

1 cup medium-grain brown rice

1 shallot, sliced

1 teaspoon salt

½ teaspoon dried oregano

¼ teaspoon freshly ground black pepper

2 cups chicken broth

1 tablespoon finely chopped fresh mint

1. In a large skillet, melt the butter over high heat.

2. Add the chicken and cook until browned, 2 to 3 minutes.

3. Add the asparagus, peas, rice, shallot, salt, oregano, and pepper and combine well.

4. Add the broth and bring to a boil.

5. Reduce the heat to a simmer, cover, and cook until the chicken and rice are tender, 20 to 30 minutes. Remove from the heat and let rest, covered, for 5 minutes.

6. Sprinkle with the mint and serve.

TIPS: *If using cooked chicken and brown rice, stir-fry the vegetables in the butter, add ½ cup of broth, and add all the remaining ingredients through the broth and stir-fry to heat through. Add the mint and serve. Store, covered, in the refrigerator for up to 5 days, or freeze for several months.*

PER SERVING Calories: 568; Total Fat: 12g; Total Carbohydrates: 78g; Sugar: 3g; Fiber: 6g; Protein: 36g; Sodium: 1068mg

STEAK AND GREEN VEGETABLES

SERVES 4 / PREP TIME: 10 MINUTES / COOK TIME: 30 MINUTES

Searing a steak over high heat and then finishing it in the oven allows for more control over desired doneness. I've used green beans and zucchini in this recipe, but the same technique can be applied using Swiss chard, spinach, or broccoli. Look for organic pastured beef. It provides better nutrition and is a more sustainable choice than regular beef.

4 (4-ounce) boneless steaks

1 tablespoon extra-virgin
   olive oil

1 teaspoon salt

¼ teaspoon freshly ground
   black pepper

2 tablespoons
   unsalted butter

1 large zucchini, cut into
   ¼-inch slices

8 ounces green beans,
   trimmed

½ cup red wine

1. Preheat the oven to 400°F.

2. Rub the steaks with the oil and season on both sides with the salt and pepper.

3. In an oven-safe skillet, melt the butter over high heat. Add the steaks and sear until golden brown, 2 to 3 minutes per side. Remove from the skillet and set aside.

4. Add the zucchini and green beans and sauté until softened, 1 to 2 minutes. Place the steaks on top of the vegetables and add the wine.

5. Transfer the skillet to the oven. Roast until the meat is cooked to your desired doneness, 10 to 15 minutes. Remove from the oven. Let rest, covered, for 5 minutes, and serve.

TIPS: *Any steak will do, but New York strip and rib-eye are both flavorful choices. Look for steaks that are 1½ to 2 inches thick. Since most steaks are larger than 4 ounces, you may want to cut them in half.*

PER SERVING Calories: 378; Total Fat: 26g; Total Carbohydrates: 7g; Sugar: 2g; Fiber: 3g; Protein: 24g; Sodium: 690mg

TURKEY AND SWEET POTATO SKILLET WITH BROCCOLI AND SHALLOT

SERVES 4 / PREP TIME: 10 MINUTES / COOK TIME: 20 MINUTES

This dish gets its quick cooking time from using the scaloppini, or thinly sliced turkey breast, available at most meat counters. Add some dried cranberries for a touch of the holidays.

2 tablespoons unsalted butter

1 shallot, thinly sliced

1 pound turkey breast cutlets

2 cups peeled sweet potatoes cut into ¼-inch dice

2 cups broccoli florets

1½ cups chicken broth

1 teaspoon salt

1 teaspoon dried sage

¼ teaspoon freshly ground black pepper

1. Preheat the oven to 400°F.

2. In an oven-safe skillet, melt the butter over high heat.

3. Add the shallot and sauté until softened, about 1 minute.

4. Add the turkey and place the sweet potatoes and broccoli on top of the turkey.

5. Add the broth and season with the salt, sage, and pepper.

6. Transfer the skillet to the oven and roast until the sweet potatoes are tender and the turkey is cooked through, about 15 minutes. Remove from the oven. Let rest, covered, for 5 minutes, and serve.

TIPS: *For a creamier sauce, replace ½ cup of chicken broth with coconut milk or unsweetened almond milk. Store, covered, for up to 5 days in the refrigerator, or freeze for several months.*

PER SERVING Calories: 261; Total Fat: 7g; Total Carbohydrates: 17g; Sugar: 4g; Fiber: 3g; Protein: 32g; Sodium: 1060mg

COD WITH LEEKS AND ZUCCHINI

SERVES 4 / PREP TIME: 10 MINUTES / COOK TIME: 25 MINUTES

Leeks are a good source of fiber, magnesium, and iron, and their delicate sweet flavor really complements the cod and zucchini.

2 tablespoons unsalted butter

2 large zucchini, cut into ¼-inch slices

2 leeks, white parts only, thinly sliced

1 garlic clove, minced

4 (4-ounce) skinless cod fillets, 1½ to 2 inches thick

1 teaspoon salt

¼ teaspoon freshly ground black pepper

½ cup white wine

1 tablespoon chopped fresh flat-leaf parsley

Lemon wedges, for serving

1. Preheat the oven to 400°F.

2. In an oven-safe skillet, melt the butter over high heat.

3. Add the zucchini, leeks, and garlic and sauté until softened and starting to brown, 3 to 4 minutes.

4. Place the cod on top of the vegetables, season with the salt and pepper, and add the wine.

5. Transfer the skillet to the oven and roast until the cod is firm, about 15 minutes. Remove from the oven and let rest, covered, for 5 minutes.

6. Sprinkle with the parsley and serve with lemon wedges.

TIPS: *Any white-fleshed fish will work in this recipe. You can even use more delicate fish like sole. If using sole, decrease the cooking time to 10 minutes. Store, covered, in the refrigerator for up to 48 hours. This dish does not freeze well.*

PER SERVING Calories: 221; Total Fat: 7g; Total Carbohydrates: 13g; Sugar: 5g; Fiber: 3g; Protein: 23g; Sodium: 730mg

SALMON WITH ASPARAGUS AND SWEET POTATOES

SERVES 4 / PREP TIME: 10 MINUTES / COOK TIME: 35 MINUTES

Not only is this dinner full of great nutrition with the omega-3s from the salmon, the vitamin B₆ and folate from the asparagus, and the vitamin A and fiber from the sweet potatoes, but also it's a colorful feast for the eyes.

2 tablespoons unsalted butter

½ red onion, finely chopped

2 cups peeled sweet potatoes cut into ¼-inch slices

1 pound skinless salmon fillets, cut into 1-inch dice

1 pound asparagus, trimmed of woody ends and cut into 1-inch pieces

1 teaspoon salt

¼ teaspoon freshly ground black pepper

½ cup white wine

Lemon wedges, for serving

1. Preheat the oven to 400°F.

2. In an oven-safe skillet, melt the butter over high heat.

3. Add the onion and sauté until softened, about 5 minutes.

4. Add the sweet potatoes and sauté until softened, 5 to 8 minutes.

5. Place the salmon and asparagus on top of the sweet potatoes. Season with the salt and pepper and add the wine.

6. Transfer the skillet to the oven. Roast until the salmon is cooked through and the asparagus is soft, 15 to 20 minutes.

7. Serve with lemon wedges.

TIPS: *You can use this technique to cook any kind of firm-fleshed fish like cod or swordfish. Store this dish, covered, in the refrigerator for up to 48 hours. This dish does not freeze well.*

PER SERVING Calories: 361; Total Fat: 18g; Total Carbohydrates: 20g; Sugar: 6g; Fiber: 5g; Protein: 26g; Sodium: 728mg

SOLE AND ZUCCHINI WITH PESTO SAUCE

SERVES 4 / PREP TIME: 10 MINUTES / COOK TIME: 15 MINUTES

Look for dairy-free or vegan pesto. Sole cooks quickly and is added at the end of the cooking time. Gluten-free pasta is a good thing to serve with this light meal.

2 tablespoons extra-virgin olive oil

2 large zucchini, cut into ¼-inch slices

1 pound sole fillets

1 teaspoon salt

½ cup white wine

¼ cup store-bought pesto

¼ teaspoon red pepper flakes (optional)

1. Preheat the oven to 400°F.

2. In an oven-safe skillet, heat the oil over high heat.

3. Add the zucchini and sauté until lightly browned, about 5 minutes.

4. Place the sole on top of the zucchini, season with the salt, and add the wine.

5. Spread the pesto over the sole and season with the red pepper flakes (if using).

6. Transfer the skillet to the oven and bake until the sole is cooked through, about 8 minutes.

TIPS: *This dish can be easily made with salmon, cod, or shrimp. If using a firm-fleshed fish, increase the cooking time accordingly. Store, covered, in the refrigerator for up to 48 hours. This dish does not freeze well.*

PER SERVING Calories: 278; Total Fat: 16g; Total Carbohydrates: 7g; Sugar: 4g; Fiber: 2g; Protein: 25g; Sodium: 784mg

SOLE WITH BROCCOLINI AND ALMONDS

SERVES 4 / PREP TIME: 10 MINUTES / COOK TIME: 20 MINUTES

Even those who don't like fish do like sole. It has a delicate flavor and cooks very quickly. This recipe gets its creaminess from unsweetened almond milk, but it can be replaced with white wine or broth.

2 tablespoons unsalted butter

2 cups broccolini cut into 2-inch pieces

2 scallions, both white and green parts, thinly sliced

½ cup unsweetened almond milk

1 teaspoon salt

¼ teaspoon freshly ground black pepper

1 pound sole fillets

¼ cup chopped fresh basil

1 tablespoon toasted slivered almonds (see tip on page 23)

1 teaspoon grated or minced lemon zest

1. Preheat the oven to 400°F.

2. In an oven-safe skillet, melt the butter over high heat.

3. Add the broccolini and scallions and sauté until softened, 2 to 3 minutes.

4. Add the almond milk, salt, and pepper.

5. Place the sole on top of the vegetables, transfer the skillet to the oven, and bake until the sole flakes with a fork and the vegetables are tender, 10 to 15 minutes.

6. Sprinkle with the basil, almonds, and lemon zest and serve.

TIPS: *This dish is delicious using just about any fish or shellfish. If using a thicker cut of fish, extend the cooking time accordingly. Store, covered, in the refrigerator for up to 48 hours. This dish does not freeze well.*

PER SERVING Calories: 185; Total Fat: 9g; Total Carbohydrates: 4g; Sugar: 1g; Fiber: 1g; Protein: 23g; Sodium: 749mg

PAN-SEARED TUNA WITH BOK CHOY

SERVES 4 / PREP TIME: 10 MINUTES / COOK TIME: 10 MINUTES

Bok choy, ginger, and sesame oil lend an Asian flavor to this dish. You do not need sushi-grade tuna for this dish, as the tuna steaks sold in the frozen seafood aisle are best. Look for steaks that are about 1 inch thick.

4 (4-ounce) tuna steaks

2 tablespoons sesame oil, divided

1 teaspoon salt

1 garlic clove, minced

1 (1¼-inch) piece fresh ginger, peeled and minced

¼ teaspoon red pepper flakes (optional)

3 cups baby bok choy cut into ½-inch pieces

1 scallion, both white and green parts, thinly sliced

2 teaspoons gluten-free tamari or soy sauce

1. Rub the tuna steaks with 1 tablespoon of sesame oil and season with the salt.

2. Heat a large skillet over high heat. When the skillet is very hot, add the steaks, and sear on both sides, leaving them still slightly rare in the middle, 2 to 3 minutes per side. Remove from the skillet.

3. Heat the remaining 1 tablespoon of sesame oil.

4. Add the garlic, ginger, and red pepper flakes (if using) and sauté until softened, about 1 minute.

5. Add the bok choy and sauté until wilted and tender, 3 to 4 minutes.

6. Return the tuna to the skillet, sprinkle with the scallion, drizzle with the tamari, and serve.

TIPS: *The best way to thaw the tuna steaks is to place them in the refrigerator overnight. Store this dish, covered, in the refrigerator for up to 48 hours. Leftovers can be added to salad for lunch. This dish should not be frozen.*

PER SERVING Calories: 191; Total Fat: 8g; Total Carbohydrates: 2g; Sugar: 1g; Fiber: 1g; Protein: 28g; Sodium: 806mg

SHRIMP AND BROCCOLINI WITH COCONUT MILK AND LEMON ZEST

SERVES 4 / PREP TIME: 10 MINUTES / COOK TIME: 10 MINUTES

This recipe uses uncooked shrimp, but you can make it with cooked shrimp if you simmer the vegetables in the sauce until tender, then add the shrimp at the end of the cooking time to warm through.

2 tablespoons extra-virgin olive oil or coconut oil

2 scallions, both white and green parts, thinly sliced

1 garlic clove, minced

1 pound peeled shrimp, thawed if necessary

2 cups broccolini cut into 1-inch pieces

1 teaspoon salt

¼ teaspoon freshly ground black pepper

1½ cups full-fat coconut milk

1 tablespoon finely chopped fresh cilantro

1 teaspoon grated or minced lemon zest

1. In a large skillet, heat the oil over high heat.

2. Add the scallions and garlic, and sauté until softened, for about 1 minute.

3. Add the shrimp, broccolini, salt, and pepper and stir to combine.

4. Add the coconut milk and simmer until the shrimp and broccolini are tender, 5 to 8 minutes.

5. Sprinkle with the cilantro and lemon zest and serve.

TIPS: *It's best to thaw frozen shrimp in the refrigerator overnight, and place in a strainer to remove the excess liquid before using. Store this dish, covered, in the refrigerator for up to 48 hours. This dish does not freeze well.*

PER SERVING Calories: 394; Total Fat: 30g; Total Carbohydrates: 9g; Sugar: 4g; Fiber: 3g; Protein: 28g; Sodium: 868mg

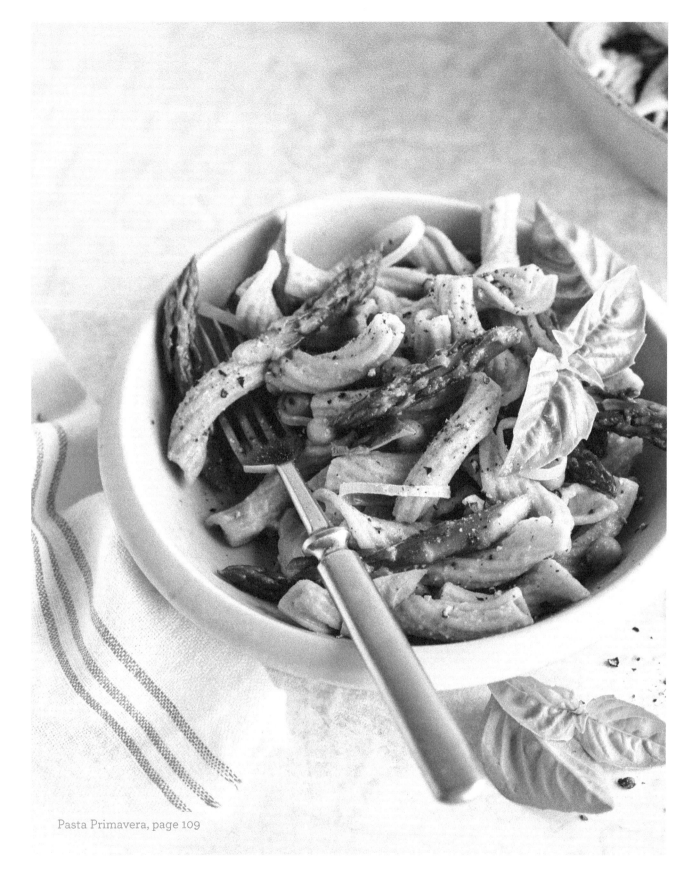

Pasta Primavera, page 109

CHAPTER 8

One-Pot Pastas

Traditionally pasta is cooked in a large pot of boiling water, drained, and added to the sauce. Most of the recipes in this chapter have been streamlined so that the entire process is done in one pot without draining the pasta. The exceptions in some cases are pastas like linguine and fettuccine or soba noodles or Asian-style rice noodles, as these more delicate noodles can easily become sticky when cooked using the one-pot cooking technique.

All the recipes in this chapter are made with gluten-free pasta, since wheat and gluten can cause inflammation. Experiment with the varieties of gluten-free pastas to see which ones you like best. Gluten-free pastas come in a variety of types, including brown rice, bean, corn, and quinoa, to name a few. We have found the best texture to come from pasta made with a corn, rice, and quinoa blend. The good news is that cooking one-pot pasta is fast and easy, and typically dinner is ready in 30 minutes or less.

MEDITERRANEAN ONE-POT PASTA

SERVES 4 / PREP TIME: 10 MINUTES / COOK TIME: 15 MINUTES

Zucchini, white beans, garlic, and oregano create the Mediterranean flavors of this pasta. Typically, this dish would have tomatoes, which can cause inflammation, so they aren't included in this dish, but the flavors are so robust, you won't miss them.

2 tablespoons extra-virgin olive oil

1 small onion, cut into ¼-inch dice

2 garlic cloves, sliced

2 small zucchini, cut into ¼-inch slices

1 teaspoon salt

1 teaspoon dried oregano

¼ teaspoon red pepper flakes (optional)

2 cups vegetable broth or water

8 ounces gluten-free penne

1 cup canned white beans

¼ cup grated sheep's milk pecorino cheese (optional)

1. In a large pot, heat the oil over high heat.

2. Add the onion and garlic and sauté until softened, 1 to 2 minutes.

3. Add the zucchini, salt, oregano, and red pepper flakes (if using) and mix well.

4. Add the broth and penne and bring to a boil. Cook, uncovered, until the penne is tender, 8 to 12 minutes.

5. Stir in the beans, sprinkle with the pecorino cheese (if using), and serve.

TIPS: *To make it vegan, omit the cheese, or if omnivorous, substitute chicken broth for vegetable broth. Store, covered, in the refrigerator for up to 5 days, or freeze for several months.*

PER SERVING Calories: 355; Total Fat: 9g; Total Carbohydrates: 59g; Sugar: 3g; Fiber: 9g; Protein: 13g; Sodium: 613mg

WINTER SQUASH AND WALNUT PASTA

SERVES 4 / PREP TIME: 10 MINUTES / COOK TIME: 15 MINUTES

This dish is typically made with whole-wheat pasta, but whole-wheat pasta has gluten and can cause inflammation, so ours is made with gluten-free pasta. Farfalle is best, but any smaller shaped pasta like orecchiette or small shells will work just as well. If you'd like to add dairy, sheep's milk feta or goat cheese is delicious with this pasta.

2 tablespoons extra-virgin olive oil, plus more for drizzling

2 cups peeled butternut squash or other winter squash cut into ¼-inch dice

½ cup diced onion

1 teaspoon salt

¼ teaspoon freshly ground black pepper

2 cups vegetable broth or water

2 cups stemmed kale leaves cut into 1-inch strips

8 ounces gluten-free farfalle

½ cup coarsely chopped toasted walnuts (see tip on page 23)

1. In a large pot, heat the oil over high heat.

2. Add the squash, onion, salt, and pepper and sauté until softened, about 2 minutes.

3. Add the broth, kale, and farfalle and bring to a boil. Cook, uncovered, until the squash and farfalle are tender, 8 to 11 minutes.

4. Ladle into bowls, sprinkle with the walnuts, drizzle with olive oil, and serve.

TIPS: *Cutting the winter squash into a ¼-inch dice is important so that the squash cooks in the same amount of time as the pasta. Store this dish, covered, in the refrigerator for up to 5 days, or freeze for several months.*

PER SERVING Calories: 343; Total Fat: 9g; Total Carbohydrates: 55g; Sugar: 4g; Fiber: 7g; Protein: 11g; Sodium: 981mg

ZUCCHINI AND PESTO PASTA

SERVES 4 / PREP TIME: 10 MINUTES / COOK TIME: 15 MINUTES

This five-ingredient pasta is one of the fastest, easiest meals to make. You can increase the protein in this dish with the addition of beans or cooked chicken. Serve garnished with grated pecorino for even more flavor.

2 tablespoons extra-virgin olive oil

2 large zucchini, cut into ¼-inch slices

2 cups vegetable broth or water

8 ounces gluten-free spaghetti

½ cup dairy-free pesto or pesto made with pecorino cheese

1. In a large pot, heat the oil over high heat.

2. Add the zucchini and sauté until softened, 2 to 3 minutes.

3. Add the broth and spaghetti and bring to a boil. Cook, uncovered, until the spaghetti is tender, 8 to 10 minutes. Drain thoroughly, then return to the pot.

4. Add the pesto, mix until combined, and serve.

TIPS: *If the pasta is watery after cooking, drain off the excess before adding the pesto. Store, covered, in the refrigerator for up to 5 days or freeze for several months. If you're unable to find dairy-free pesto, make it easily by combining ¼ cup pine nuts (or almonds), 3 tablespoons extra-virgin olive oil, 2 tablespoons chopped fresh basil, 1 garlic clove, 2 teaspoons lemon juice, and ¼ teaspoon salt in a food processor. Pulse until finely ground. This will make enough for this recipe, about ½ cup.*

PER SERVING Calories: 431; Total Fat: 22g; Total Carbohydrates: 48g; Sugar: 6g; Fiber: 7g; Protein: 12g; Sodium: 206mg

SPAGHETTI WITH ALMONDS, MINT, AND FETA

SERVES 4 / PREP TIME: 10 MINUTES / COOK TIME: 15 MINUTES

Fava beans and mint go well together. Some markets sell frozen fava beans. If they aren't available in your market, substitute frozen peas or lima beans.

2 tablespoons extra-virgin olive oil

½ onion, minced

2 cups vegetable broth or water

1 (10-ounce) bag frozen fava beans, thawed

8 ounces gluten-free spaghetti

1 teaspoon salt

¼ teaspoon freshly ground black pepper

½ cup ground almonds

1 tablespoon finely chopped fresh mint

½ cup crumbled sheep's or goat's milk feta cheese

1. In a large pot, heat the oil over high heat.

2. Add the onion and sauté until softened, 1 to 2 minutes.

3. Add the broth, fava beans, spaghetti, salt, and pepper and bring to a boil. Cook, uncovered, until the spaghetti is tender, about 10 minutes.

4. Add the almonds and mint and mix well.

5. Sprinkle with the cheese and serve.

TIPS: *Cooked chicken or shrimp is a good addition to this recipe. Store this dish, covered, in the refrigerator for up to 5 days, or freeze for several months.*

PER SERVING Calories: 393; Total Fat: 12g; Total Carbohydrates: 57g; Sugar: 2g; Fiber: 9g; Protein: 51g; Sodium: 721mg

WHITE BEAN, RED ONION, AND LEMON ZEST PASTA

SERVES 4 / PREP TIME: 10 MINUTES / COOK TIME: 15 MINUTES

Leftovers can be splashed with olive oil and lemon juice and served as a salad atop a bed of greens.

2 tablespoons extra-virgin olive oil, plus more for drizzling

1 small red onion, thinly sliced

1 garlic clove, minced

2 cups vegetable broth or water

8 ounces gluten-free rotini

1 teaspoon salt

¼ teaspoon red pepper flakes (optional)

1 cup canned white beans, drained and rinsed

2 teaspoons grated or minced lemon zest

2 teaspoons finely chopped fresh rosemary

1. In a large pot, heat the oil over high heat.

2. Add the onion and garlic and sauté until softened, 1 to 2 minutes.

3. Add the broth, rotini, salt, and red pepper flakes (if using) and bring to a boil. Cook, uncovered, until the rotini is tender, about 10 minutes.

4. Add the beans, lemon zest, and rosemary and mix well.

5. Serve drizzled with additional olive oil.

TIPS: *Walnut oil and hazelnut oil are both delicious in this recipe instead of olive oil. Nut oils are minimally processed and full of healthy fats and vitamins. They are costly and should be stored in the refrigerator and used within several months of opening. Store this dish, covered, in the refrigerator for up to 5 days, or freeze for several months.*

PER SERVING Calories: 364; Total Fat: 10g; Total Carbohydrates: 56g; Sugar: 2g; Fiber: 11g; Protein: 14g; Sodium: 964mg

PASTA PRIMAVERA

SERVES 4 / PREP TIME: 10 MINUTES / COOK TIME: 20 MINUTES

Primavera is Italian for "spring," and this pasta dish is bursting with spring vegetables. We like to use asparagus, peas, and leek when we make it, but any vegetables will do. Traditionally the sauce is a white wine cream sauce, and in this version, goat cheese adds the creaminess.

2 tablespoons unsalted butter

1 leek, white part only, thinly sliced

1 pound pencil-thin asparagus, trimmed of woody ends and cut into ½-inch pieces

1 cup frozen green peas, thawed

1 teaspoon salt

¼ teaspoon freshly ground black pepper

½ cup white wine

2 cups vegetable broth or water

8 ounces gluten-free ziti

½ cup crumbled goat cheese cheese

2 tablespoons finely chopped fresh basil

1. In a large pot, melt the butter over high heat.

2. Add the leek, asparagus, peas, salt, and pepper and sauté until softened, 1 to 2 minutes.

3. Add the wine and cook until it is reduced by half, 3 to 5 minutes.

4. Add the broth and ziti and bring to a boil. Cook, uncovered, until the ziti is tender, 10 to 12 minutes.

5. Add the cheese and stir until it melts into the ziti.

6. Sprinkle with the basil and serve.

TIPS: *Sheep's milk ricotta is a good substitute for the goat cheese in this recipe. It can be found at gourmet or farmers' markets. Store this dish, covered, in the refrigerator for up to 5 days. This dish does not freeze well.*

PER SERVING Calories: 409; Total Fat: 11g; Total Carbohydrates: 55g; Sugar: 7g; Fiber: 10g; Protein: 17g; Sodium: 1066mg

COCONUT CURRY PASTA

SERVES 4 / PREP TIME: 10 MINUTES / COOK TIME: 15 MINUTES

Brown rice noodles are the gluten-free pasta used in this recipe, which is more a soup than pasta. If you can't find them, 100-percent buckwheat soba noodles or any other gluten-free pasta will work.

8 ounces brown rice
   noodles

1 tablespoon coconut oil

½ red onion, minced

1 garlic clove, minced

1 teaspoon curry powder

1 teaspoon salt

¼ teaspoon freshly ground
   black pepper

4 cups baby spinach

1 large zucchini, thinly sliced

1 (13½-ounce) can full-fat
   coconut milk

1 cup snow peas

1 cup vegetable broth

1 scallion, both white and
   green parts, thinly sliced

1 tablespoon finely
   chopped fresh cilantro

1. Bring a large pot of water to a boil.

2. Add the rice noodles and cook according to the package directions until al dente. Drain thoroughly and set aside.

3. Melt the coconut oil over high heat.

4. Add the onion and garlic and sauté until softened, 1 to 2 minutes.

5. Add the curry powder, salt, and pepper and sauté to toast the spices, about 1 minute.

6. Add the spinach, zucchini, coconut milk, snow peas, and broth and bring to a boil.

7. Reduce the heat to a simmer and cook until the zucchini is tender, about 5 minutes.

8. Add the noodles, scallion, and cilantro, mix well, and serve.

TIPS: *Use any vegetables you'd like for this dish. Soft vegetables like zucchini, greens, and peas are best since they cook quickly. Store, covered, in the refrigerator for up to 5 days, or freeze for several months.*

PER SERVING Calories: 435; Total Fat: 29g; Total Carbohydrates: 40g; Sugar: 9g; Fiber: 6g; Protein: 9g; Sodium: 928mg

SOBA NOODLES WITH TOFU AND VEGETABLES

SERVES 4 / PREP TIME: 10 MINUTES / COOK TIME: 10 MINUTES

Look for soba noodles made entirely of buckwheat, which despite having the word "wheat" in it, isn't wheat, but rather a grain-like seed. Buckwheat is a good source of protein and fiber.

3 cups vegetable broth

8 ounces soba noodles

1 cup shredded carrots

1 cup broccoli florets

1 cup snow peas

1 tablespoon honey

1 garlic clove, minced

8 ounces firm tofu, cut into
½-inch dice

2 teaspoons sesame oil

2 teaspoons rice vinegar

2 teaspoons gluten-free
tamari or soy sauce

1. In a large pot, bring the broth to a boil.

2. Add the noodles, carrots, broccoli, snow peas, honey, and garlic and return to a boil. Cook, uncovered, until the noodles are tender, 7 to 8 minutes.

3. Add the tofu, oil, vinegar, and tamari. Stir to combine, and serve.

TIPS: *Packaged shredded carrots and broccoli florets are sold at many grocery stores in the produce department. Store this dish, covered, in the refrigerator for up to 5 days, or freeze for several months.*

PER SERVING Calories: 335; Total Fat: 6g; Total Carbohydrates: 56g; Sugar: 9g; Fiber: 3g; Protein: 19g; Sodium: 1206mg

CHICKEN AND BUTTERNUT SQUASH PASTA WITH SAGE

SERVES 4 / PREP TIME: 15 MINUTES / COOK TIME: 20 MINUTES

A hearty pasta like ziti or penne is best for this dish, as its firm texture can stand up to the chicken and butternut squash. Feel free to use any winter squash you'd like, and if you like your pasta creamy, garnish with goat cheese.

2 tablespoons unsalted butter

1 small onion, cut into ¼-inch dice

8 ounces boneless, skinless chicken breast, cut into ½-inch pieces

1 teaspoon salt

¼ teaspoon freshly ground black pepper

⅛ teaspoon ground nutmeg

2 cups peeled butternut squash cut into ¼-inch dice

2 cups chicken or vegetable broth

8 ounces gluten-free ziti

2 teaspoons finely chopped fresh sage

1. In a large pot, melt the butter over high heat.

2. Add the onion and sauté until softened, about 1 minute.

3. Add the chicken, salt, pepper, and nutmeg and sauté to lightly brown the chicken, about 3 minutes.

4. Add the squash, broth, and ziti and bring to a boil. Cook, uncovered, until the ziti is tender, 10 to 12 minutes.

5. Sprinkle with the sage and serve.

TIPS: *Many markets sell diced butternut squash in the produce section. Store this dish, covered, in the refrigerator for up to 5 days, or freeze for several months.*

PER SERVING Calories: 471; Total Fat: 11g; Total Carbohydrates: 51g; Sugar: 3g; Fiber: 7g; Protein: 40g; Sodium: 699mg

BEEF AND MUSHROOM PASTA

SERVES 4 / PREP TIME: 10 MINUTES / COOK TIME: 20 MINUTES

Think of this as a sort of "hamburger helper." Ground beef, mushrooms, and onion are cooked with elbow macaroni and topped with grated pecorino cheese. If possible, purchase organic grass-fed ground beef.

1 tablespoon unsalted butter

1 cup thinly sliced mushrooms

½ onion, finely chopped

8 ounces ground beef

1 teaspoon salt

½ teaspoon dried oregano

¼ teaspoon freshly ground black pepper

2 cups chicken broth or water

8 ounces gluten-free elbow macaroni

¼ cup grated sheep's milk pecorino cheese

1. In a large pot, melt the butter over high heat.

2. Add the mushrooms and onion and sauté until the softened, about 3 minutes.

3. Crumble the ground beef into the pot, and add the salt, oregano, and pepper.

4. Cook the beef until browned on all sides, 3 to 4 minutes total. If desired, drain any extra fat that may accumulate in the pot.

5. Add the broth and macaroni and bring to a boil. Cook, uncovered, until the macaroni is tender, about 8 minutes.

6. Sprinkle with the cheese and serve.

TIPS: *This dish can be made with ground turkey, chicken, or lamb instead of the ground beef. Store this dish, covered, for up to 5 days in the refrigerator, or freeze for several months.*

PER SERVING Calories: 370; Total Fat: 11g; Total Carbohydrates: 44g; Sugar: 2g; Fiber: 6g; Protein: 23g; Sodium: 1168mg

PASTA WITH ANCHOVIES AND SPINACH

SERVES 4 / PREP TIME: 10 MINUTES / COOK TIME: 20 MINUTES

Traditionally anchovies come in tins packed in oil and can be quite salty. For milder anchovies, look for water-packed tins. Anchovies are an excellent source of omega-3 fats and proteins.

2 tablespoons extra-virgin olive oil, plus more for drizzling

1 garlic clove, minced

4 cups baby spinach

2 cups vegetable broth or water

8 ounces gluten-free pasta

2 (4.4-ounce) cans anchovies, drained

1 teaspoon grated or minced lemon zest

1. In a large pot, heat the oil over high heat.

2. Add the garlic and sauté until softened, 1 to 2 minutes.

3. Add the spinach and cook until wilted, about 1 minute.

4. Add the broth and pasta and bring to a boil. Cook, uncovered, until the pasta is tender, 8 to 11 minutes.

5. Add the anchovies and lemon zest and combine well.

6. Drizzle with olive oil and serve.

TIPS: *There's no added salt in this recipe. If using unsalted water-packed anchovies, you may want to add ½ teaspoon of salt to the recipe. Store, covered, in the refrigerator for up to 3 days, or freeze for several months.*

PER SERVING Calories: 416; Total Fat: 15g; Total Carbohydrates: 42g; Sugar: 2g; Fiber: 6g; Protein: 27g; Sodium: 1865mg

RIGATONI WITH SARDINES, BROCCOLINI, AND GREEN OLIVES

SERVES 4 / PREP TIME: 10 MINUTES / COOK TIME: 20 MINUTES

Sardines and olives provide an intense salty flavor, so no additional salt is needed. If possible, use broccolini in this dish, since it cooks quickly. Choose a hearty pasta like rigatoni, penne, or ziti for this recipe.

2 tablespoons extra-virgin olive oil, plus more for drizzling

2 cups broccolini cut into ½-inch pieces

1 garlic clove, minced

¼ teaspoon red pepper flakes (optional)

2½ cups vegetable broth or water

8 ounces rigatoni

1 (6-ounce) can sardines, drained

½ cup coarsely chopped pitted green olives

1. In a large pot, heat the oil over high heat.

2. Add the broccolini, garlic, and red pepper flakes (if using) and sauté until the garlic is fragrant, about 2 minutes.

3. Add the broth and rigatoni and bring to a boil. Cook, uncovered, until the rigatoni is tender, 10 to 12 minutes.

4. Add the sardines and olives and combine well.

5. Drizzle with oil and serve.

TIPS: *Anchovies can be substituted for the sardines, and if you like a milder flavor, use water-packed anchovies. Store this dish, covered, in the refrigerator for up to 5 days, or freeze for several months.*

PER SERVING Calories: 378; Total Fat: 16g; Total Carbohydrates: 49g; Sugar: 3g; Fiber: 4g; Protein: 9g; Sodium: 1163mg

SPAGHETTI WITH SHRIMP, ASPARAGUS, AND GARLIC

SERVES 4 / PREP TIME: 10 MINUTES / COOK TIME: 20 MINUTES

This pasta has all the classic flavors of scampi: butter, garlic, and white wine. We've added asparagus to this recipe, but feel free to substitute any seasonal vegetable you like.

2 tablespoons unsalted butter

4 large mushrooms, sliced

2 garlic cloves, thinly sliced

¼ cup white wine

1 pound peeled shrimp, thawed if necessary

2 cups vegetable broth or water

8 ounces gluten-free spaghetti

1 teaspoon salt

¼ teaspoon freshly ground black pepper

1 pound pencil-thin asparagus, trimmed of woody ends and cut into 1-inch pieces

1 tablespoon finely chopped fresh flat-leaf parsley

1. In a large pot, melt the butter over high heat.

2. Add the mushrooms and garlic and sauté until softened, about 3 minutes.

3. Add the wine and cook until evaporated, 2 to 3 minutes.

4. Add the shrimp, broth, spaghetti, salt, and pepper and bring to a boil. Cook, uncovered, for 4 minutes.

5. Add the asparagus and return to a boil. Cook, uncovered, until the spaghetti is tender, 4 to 6 minutes.

6. Sprinkle with the parsley and serve.

TIPS: *When using thinner gluten-free pastas like spaghetti, fettuccine, or angel hair, test them after 5 minutes, since they may cook faster than expected. Store this dish, covered, in the refrigerator, and eat within 48 hours. This dish does not freeze well.*

PER SERVING Calories: 431; Total Fat: 10g; Total Carbohydrates: 48g; Sugar: 4g; Fiber: 8g; Protein: 37g; Sodium: 1265mg

LINGUINE WITH CLAM SAUCE

SERVES 4 / PREP TIME: 10 MINUTES / COOK TIME: 20 MINUTES

This recipe is an exception to most of the recipes in this chapter, since the linguine is cooked in the traditional way, in a large pot of boiling water, and drained. While the linguine drains, the sauce is quickly prepared, then the pasta is returned to the pot to combine the flavors.

8 ounces gluten-free linguine

2 tablespoons unsalted butter

1 (10-ounce) can whole clams

½ cup white wine

1 garlic clove, minced

½ teaspoon salt

¼ teaspoon red pepper flakes (optional)

1 tablespoon finely chopped fresh flat-leaf parsley

1. Bring a large pot of water to a boil.

2. Add the linguine and cook according to the package directions until al dente. Drain thoroughly and set aside.

3. Melt the butter over medium heat.

4. Add the clams and their juices, wine, garlic, salt, and red pepper flakes (if using) and bring to a boil.

5. Return the linguine to the pot and stir to coat with the sauce.

6. Sprinkle with the parsley and serve.

TIPS: *Because linguine is thinner than spaghetti, it is more likely to get sticky if cooked in a pot with the other ingredients like many of the other recipes are. Store, covered, in the refrigerator for up to 48 hours. This dish does not freeze well.*

PER SERVING Calories: 308; Total Fat: 8g; Total Carbohydrates: 44g; Sugar: 1g; Fiber: 2g; Protein: 11g; Sodium: 513mg

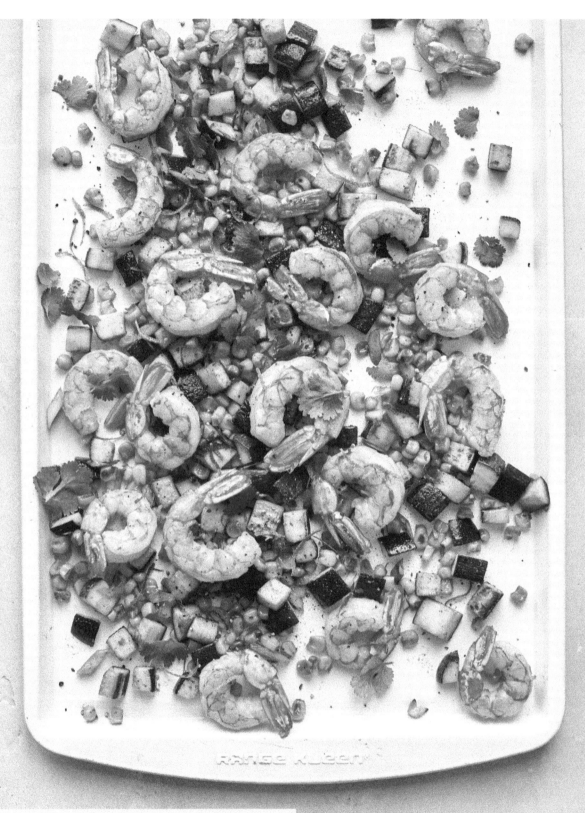

Shrimp-Lime Bake with Zucchini and Corn, page 133

CHAPTER 9

Sheet Pan Suppers

Sheet pan suppers are fast, easy, and very low tech. All that is needed is a rimmed baking sheet, delicious ingredients, and an oven, and in short order, dinner is done! The best technique for all-in-one cooking on a sheet pan is to start by putting the items in the oven that will need the longest amount of time to cook first. Then, add the remaining ingredients after 10 or 15 minutes, so that everything will be done at the same time, and nothing will be overcooked. Since baking sheets have a lot of surface area, they brown and caramelize the food well, adding deeper flavor to the dish. It's easy to cook double batches on a baking sheet so that there are leftovers for workweek lunches.

ROASTED VEGETABLES WITH SWEET POTATOES AND WHITE BEANS

SERVES 4 / PREP TIME: 15 MINUTES / COOK TIME: 25 MINUTES

Feel free to "cheat" with this recipe, and use roasted vegetables and sweet potatoes from the market salad bar. If using already cooked vegetables, you can throw this in the oven to heat through and be eating in about 10 minutes.

2 small sweet potatoes, peeled and cut into ½-inch dice

½ red onion, cut into ¼-inch dice

1 medium carrot, peeled and thinly sliced

4 ounces green beans, trimmed

¼ cup extra-virgin olive oil

1 teaspoon salt

¼ teaspoon freshly ground black pepper

1 (15½-ounce) can white beans, drained and rinsed

1 tablespoon minced or grated lemon zest

1 tablespoon chopped fresh dill

1. Preheat the oven to 400°F.

2. On a large rimmed baking sheet, combine the sweet potatoes, onion, carrot, green beans, oil, salt, and pepper and mix to combine well. Arrange in a single layer.

3. Transfer the baking sheet to the oven and roast until the vegetables are tender, 20 to 25 minutes.

4. Add the white beans, lemon zest, and dill, mix well, and serve.

TIPS: *When cooking a lot of different ingredients at the same time, it's best to try to cut all the food into the same-size pieces. The smaller the pieces, the faster they will cook. Feel free to substitute any seasonal vegetables you like. Store, covered, in the refrigerator for up to 5 days, or freeze for several months.*

PER SERVING Calories: 315; Total Fat: 13g; Total Carbohydrates: 42g; Sugar: 5g; Fiber: 13g; Protein: 10g; Sodium: 632mg

ROASTED TOFU AND GREENS

SERVES 4 / PREP TIME: 10 MINUTES / COOK TIME: 20 MINUTES

The greens are "sautéed" in the oven first, then the tofu is added over the greens and placed in the oven to roast. Tofu is a flavor sponge, so it will absorb the flavors of the ginger, garlic, and sesame oil. This is great served over brown rice.

3 cups baby spinach or kale

1 tablespoon sesame oil

1 tablespoon minced or grated peeled fresh ginger

1 garlic clove, minced

1 pound firm tofu, cut into 1-inch dice

1 tablespoon gluten-free tamari or soy sauce

¼ teaspoon red pepper flakes (optional)

1 teaspoon rice vinegar

2 scallions, both white and green parts, thinly sliced

1. Preheat the oven to 400°F.

2. On a large rimmed baking sheet, combine the spinach, oil, ginger, and garlic.

3. Transfer the baking sheet to the oven and bake until the spinach has wilted, 3 to 5 minutes.

4. Add the tofu, tamari, and red pepper flakes (if using) and toss to combine well.

5. Return the baking sheet to the oven and bake until the tofu is beginning to brown, 10 to 15 minutes.

6. Top with the vinegar and scallions and serve.

TIPS: *If tofu is hard to digest, try tempeh instead. The fermentation makes it more digestible for some people. Store this dish, covered, in the refrigerator for up to 5 days. This dish does not freeze well.*

PER SERVING Calories: 121; Total Fat: 8g; Total Carbohydrates: 4g; Sugar: 1g; Fiber: 2g; Protein: 10g; Sodium: 258mg

TOFU AND ITALIAN-SEASONED SUMMER VEGETABLES

SERVES 4 / PREP TIME: 10 MINUTES / COOK TIME: 20 MINUTES

We love this recipe because it's so easy. Arrange seasonal vegetables and tofu in the pan, and generously season with Italian herbs and you're done. Serve with brown rice for a complete meal.

2 large zucchini, cut into ¼-inch slices

2 large summer squash, cut into ¼-inch-thick slices

1 pound firm tofu, cut into 1-inch dice

1 cup vegetable broth or water

3 tablespoons extra-virgin olive oil

2 garlic cloves, sliced

1 teaspoon salt

1 teaspoon Italian herb seasoning blend

¼ teaspoon freshly ground black pepper

1 tablespoon thinly sliced fresh basil

1. Preheat the oven to 400°F.

2. On a large rimmed baking sheet, combine the zucchini, squash, tofu, broth, oil, garlic, salt, Italian herb seasoning blend, and pepper and mix well.

3. Transfer the baking sheet to the oven and roast until the squash is tender and the tofu is lightly browned, about 20 minutes.

4. Sprinkle with the basil and serve.

TIPS: *Chickpeas or white beans can be substituted for tofu in this dish. Leftovers can be combined with vegetable broth to create a delicious soup. Store, covered, in the refrigerator for up to 5 days, or freeze for several months.*

PER SERVING Calories: 213; Total Fat: 16g; Total Carbohydrates: 9g; Sugar: 4g; Fiber: 3g; Protein: 13g; Sodium: 806mg

SPICED BROCCOLI, CAULIFLOWER, AND TOFU WITH RED ONION

SERVES 4 / PREP TIME: 10 MINUTES / COOK TIME: 25 MINUTES

Many markets sell broccoli and cauliflower florets, which eliminates the need to cut the vegetables. Roasting cruciferous vegetables will make even those who don't like vegetables eat them, as it makes them sweet and crunchy.

2 cups broccoli florets

2 cups cauliflower florets

1 medium red onion, diced

3 tablespoons extra-virgin olive oil

1 teaspoon salt

¼ teaspoon freshly ground black pepper

1 pound firm tofu, cut into 1-inch dice

1 garlic clove, minced

1 (¼-inch) piece fresh ginger, minced

1. Preheat the oven to 400°F.

2. On a large rimmed baking sheet, combine the broccoli, cauliflower, onion, oil, salt, and pepper and mix well.

3. Transfer the baking sheet to the oven and roast until the vegetables have softened, 10 to 15 minutes.

4. Add the tofu, garlic, and ginger.

5. Return the baking sheet to the oven and roast until the vegetables are tender and the tofu is lightly browned, about 10 minutes.

6. Gently mix the ingredients on the baking sheet to combine the tofu with the vegetables and serve.

TIPS: *If you're avoiding soy, you can make this dish with canned beans or cooked chicken. Store, covered, in the refrigerator for up to 5 days, or freeze for several months.*

PER SERVING Calories: 210; Total Fat: 15g; Total Carbohydrates: 11g; Sugar: 4g; Fiber: 4g; Protein: 12g; Sodium: 626mg

TEMPEH AND ROOT VEGETABLE BAKE

SERVES 4 / PREP TIME: 10 MINUTES / COOK TIME: 30 MINUTES

Tempeh is a fermented soy product and is typically found where all the vegetarian proteins are sold. It can come in many flavors, which will be fun to experiment with when making this recipe. Enjoy with brown rice or quinoa.

1 tablespoon extra-virgin olive oil or coconut oil

1 large sweet potato, peeled and cut into ¼-inch dice

2 carrots, thinly sliced

1 fennel bulb, trimmed and cut into ¼-inch dice

2 teaspoons minced fresh ginger

1 garlic clove, minced

12 ounces tempeh, cut into ½-inch dice

½ cup vegetable broth

1 tablespoon gluten-free tamari or soy sauce

2 scallions, both white and green parts, thinly sliced

1. Preheat the oven to 400°F. Coat a large rimmed baking sheet with the oil.

2. Arrange the sweet potato, carrots, fennel, ginger, and garlic in a single layer on the baking sheet.

3. Transfer the baking sheet to the oven and bake until the vegetables have softened, about 15 minutes.

4. Add the tempeh, broth, and tamari.

5. Return the baking sheet to the oven and bake until the tempeh is heated through and lightly browned, 10 to 15 minutes.

6. Add the scallions, mix well, and serve.

TIPS: *If you can't find tempeh, substitute tofu. Store this dish, covered, in the refrigerator for up to 5 days. This dish does not freeze well.*

PER SERVING Calories: 276; Total Fat: 13g; Total Carbohydrates: 26g; Sugar: 5g; Fiber: 4g; Protein: 19g; Sodium: 397mg

GARLICKY CHICKEN AND VEGETABLES

SERVES 4 / PREP TIME: 10 MINUTES / COOK TIME: 45 MINUTES

Chicken on the bone with skin is the best chicken for this recipe, since it has the most flavor.

2 teaspoons extra-virgin olive oil

1 leek, white part only, thinly sliced

2 large zucchini, cut into ¼-inch slices

4 bone-in, skin-on chicken breasts

3 garlic cloves, minced

1 teaspoon salt

1 teaspoon dried oregano

¼ teaspoon freshly ground black pepper

½ cup white wine

Juice of 1 lemon

1. Preheat the oven to 400°F. Coat a large rimmed baking sheet with the oil.

2. Place the leek and zucchini on the baking sheet.

3. Place the chicken, skin-side up, on top of the vegetables and sprinkle with the garlic, salt, oregano, and pepper. Add the wine.

4. Transfer the baking sheet to the oven and roast until the chicken is golden and cooked through, 35 to 40 minutes. Remove from the oven and let rest for 5 minutes.

5. Add the lemon juice and serve.

TIPS: *If using boneless, skinless chicken breast, coat it with some of the olive oil before roasting; this will help it brown. Store, covered, in the refrigerator for up to 5 days, or freeze for several months.*

PER SERVING Calories: 315; Total Fat: 8g; Total Carbohydrates: 12g; Sugar: 4g; Fiber: 2g; Protein: 44g; Sodium: 685mg

TURMERIC-SPICED SWEET POTATOES, APPLE, AND ONION WITH CHICKEN

SERVES 4 / PREP TIME: 15 MINUTES / COOK TIME: 45 MINUTES

The flavors in this dish provide a little bit of the holidays throughout the year. You can make this with a half boneless turkey breast, and serve with cranberry sauce to increase the comfort food level.

2 tablespoons unsalted butter, at room temperature

2 medium sweet potatoes, peeled and cut into ¼-inch slices

1 large Granny Smith apple, cored and cut into ¼-inch slices

1 medium onion, thinly sliced

4 bone-in, skin-on chicken breasts

1 teaspoon salt

1 teaspoon turmeric

1 teaspoon dried sage

¼ teaspoon freshly ground black pepper

1 cup apple cider, white wine, or chicken broth

1. Preheat the oven to 400°F. Coat a large rimmed baking sheet with the butter.

2. Arrange the sweet potatoes, apple, and onion in a single layer on the baking sheet.

3. Place the chicken on top of the vegetables, skin-side up, and season with the salt, turmeric, sage, and pepper. Add the cider.

4. Transfer the baking sheet to the oven, and roast until the chicken is cooked and the vegetables are tender, 35 to 40 minutes. Remove from the oven, let rest for 5 minutes, and serve.

TIPS: *If using boneless turkey breast, the cooking time will increase to 45 to 55 minutes. Store, covered, in the refrigerator for up to 5 days, or freeze for several months.*

PER SERVING Calories: 386; Total Fat: 12g; Total Carbohydrates: 26g; Sugar: 10g; Fiber: 4g; Protein: 44g; Sodium: 932mg

HONEY-ROASTED CHICKEN THIGHS WITH CARROTS

SERVES 4 / PREP TIME: 10 MINUTES / COOK TIME: 50 MINUTES

This recipe uses chicken thighs with the bone, but if saving time is the name of the game, boneless thighs will cook quicker. Serve with quinoa for a complete meal.

2 tablespoons unsalted butter, at room temperature

3 large carrots, thinly sliced

2 garlic cloves, minced

4 bone-in, skin-on chicken thighs

1 teaspoon salt

½ teaspoon dried rosemary

¼ teaspoon freshly ground black pepper

2 tablespoons honey

1 cup chicken broth or vegetable broth

Lemon wedges, for serving

1. Preheat the oven to 400°F. Coat a large rimmed baking sheet with the butter.

2. Arrange the carrots and garlic in a single layer on the baking sheet.

3. Place the chicken, skin-side up, on top of the vegetables, and season with the salt, rosemary, and pepper.

4. Drizzle the honey on top and add the broth.

5. Transfer the baking sheet to the oven and roast until the chicken is cooked through and the carrots are tender, 40 to 45 minutes. Remove from the oven, let rest for 5 minutes, and serve with lemon wedges.

TIPS: *Boneless chicken breast can be substituted for chicken thighs, but it will decrease the cooking time to around 25 minutes. Store, covered, in the refrigerator for up to 5 days. This dish does not freeze well.*

PER SERVING Calories: 428; Total Fat: 28g; Total Carbohydrates: 15g; Sugar: 11g; Fiber: 2g; Protein: 30g; Sodium: 732mg

SESAME-TAMARI BAKED CHICKEN WITH GREEN BEANS

SERVES 4 / PREP TIME: 10 MINUTES / COOK TIME: 45 MINUTES

Sesame oil, tamari, and honey glaze this chicken, which is sitting on a bed of green beans. This family favorite recipe is great served with brown rice.

1 pound green beans, trimmed

4 bone-in, skin-on chicken breasts

2 tablespoons honey

1 tablespoon sesame oil

1 tablespoon gluten-free tamari or soy sauce

1 cup chicken or vegetable broth

1. Preheat the oven to 400°F.

2. Arrange the green beans in a single layer on a large rimmed baking sheet.

3. Place the chicken, skin-side up, on top of the beans.

4. Drizzle with the honey, oil, and tamari. Add the broth.

5. Transfer the baking sheet to the oven and roast until the chicken is cooked through and the vegetables are tender, 35 to 40 minutes. Remove from the oven, let rest for 5 minutes, and serve.

TIPS: *Any seasonal vegetable can be substituted for the green beans. Asparagus and zucchini are good options. Store this dish, covered, in the refrigerator for up to 5 days, or freeze for several months.*

PER SERVING Calories: 378; Total Fat: 10g; Total Carbohydrates: 19g; Sugar: 10g; Fiber: 4g; Protein: 54g; Sodium: 336mg

SHEET PAN TURKEY BREAST WITH GOLDEN VEGETABLES

SERVES 4 / PREP TIME: 15 MINUTES / COOK TIME: 50 MINUTES

A boneless half turkey breast is best for this recipe, since it will cook quickly. The golden vegetables in this dish deliciously provide antioxidants.

2 tablespoons unsalted butter, at room temperature

1 medium acorn squash, seeded and thinly sliced

2 large golden beets, peeled and thinly sliced

½ medium yellow onion, thinly sliced

½ boneless, skin-on turkey breast (1 to 2 pounds)

2 tablespoons honey

1 teaspoon salt

1 teaspoon turmeric

¼ teaspoon freshly ground black pepper

1 cup chicken broth or vegetable broth

1. Preheat the oven to 400°F. Coat a large rimmed baking sheet with the butter.

2. Arrange the squash, beets, and onion in a single layer on the baking sheet. Place the turkey, skin-side up, on top of the vegetables. Drizzle with the honey. Season with the salt, turmeric, and pepper, and add the broth.

3. Transfer the baking sheet to the oven and roast until the turkey registers 165°F in the center with an instant-read thermometer, 35 to 45 minutes. Remove from the oven and let rest for 5 minutes.

4. Slice the turkey and serve with the vegetables and pan juices.

TIPS: *Boneless turkey breasts with skin on are found at most markets and can range widely in size. You may see entire turkey breasts, or half breasts; for this recipe a half breast is plenty to serve four. You will most likely have leftover turkey meat, which can be used in salads or soups. Store this dish, covered, in the refrigerator for up to 5 days. This dish does not freeze well.*

PER SERVING Calories: 383; Total Fat: 15g; Total Carbohydrates: 25g; Sugar: 13g; Fiber: 3g; Protein: 37g; Sodium: 748mg

SHEET PAN STEAK WITH BRUSSELS SPROUTS AND RED WINE

SERVES 4 / PREP TIME: 10 MINUTES / COOK TIME: 20 MINUTES

In order to get a good char on the steak, it's started in the broiler and finished in the oven.

1 pound rib eye steak

1 teaspoon salt

¼ teaspoon freshly ground black pepper

1 tablespoon unsalted butter

½ red onion, minced

8 ounces Brussels sprouts, trimmed and quartered

1 cup red wine

Juice of ½ lemon

1. Preheat the broiler on high.

2. On a large rimmed baking sheet, season the steak with the salt and pepper. Broil until browned, 2 to 3 minutes per side.

3. Turn off the broiler and preheat the oven to 400°F.

4. Place the steak on one side of the baking sheet and add the butter, onion, Brussels sprouts, and wine to the other side.

5. Transfer the baking sheet to the oven and roast until the steak is cooked to your desired doneness and the Brussels sprouts are tender, about 8 minutes. Remove from the oven and let rest for 5 minutes. (If the steak cooks faster than the sprouts, remove it from the oven, spread the sprouts in the baking sheet, and return to the oven until tender.)

6. Sprinkle with the lemon juice and serve.

TIPS: *The recipe calls for rib-eye, but a New York strip will work just as well. Store this dish, covered, in the refrigerator for up to 5 days. This dish does not freeze well.*

PER SERVING Calories: 416; Total Fat: 27g; Total Carbohydrates: 8g; Sugar: 2g; Fiber: 3g; Protein: 22g; Sodium: 636mg

MISO SALMON AND GREEN BEANS

SERVES 4 / PREP TIME: 10 MINUTES / COOK TIME: 25 MINUTES

Miso is a fermented soybean paste, but it can also be made with other ingredients. We've used white miso in this recipe, since its delicate flavor goes well with salmon. Miso is rich in essential minerals and B vitamins, and since it's a fermented product, it aids in digestion.

1 tablespoon sesame oil

1 pound green beans, trimmed

1 pound skin-on salmon fillets, cut into 4 steaks

¼ cup white miso

2 teaspoons gluten-free tamari or soy sauce

2 scallions, both white and green parts, thinly sliced

1. Preheat the oven to 400°F. Coat a large rimmed baking sheet with the oil.

2. Arrange the green beans in a single layer on the baking sheet.

3. Place the salmon on top of the green beans and brush each piece with the miso.

4. Transfer the baking sheet to the oven and roast until the salmon is cooked through and the green beans are tender, 20 to 25 minutes.

5. Drizzle with the tamari, sprinkle with the scallions, and serve.

TIPS: *Miso can be sold either in the refrigerated soy product section of the store, or on the shelves where other Asian products are sold. Once open, it should be refrigerated but has a very long shelf life. It's good to have on hand for quick miso soup. All that is needed is to add water or broth. The salmon can be stored, covered, in the refrigerator for up to 48 hours. This dish does not freeze well.*

PER SERVING Calories: 213; Total Fat: 7g; Total Carbohydrates: 13g; Sugar: 3g; Fiber: 5g; Protein: 27g; Sodium: 989mg

TILAPIA WITH ASPARAGUS AND ACORN SQUASH

SERVES 4 / PREP TIME: 15 MINUTES / COOK TIME: 30 MINUTES

The acorn squash can be prepared in two ways, either very thinly sliced, or in ¼-inch wedges. In both preparations, there's no need to peel, since the roasted skin can be eaten. Any firm-fleshed fish can be substituted for the tilapia.

2 tablespoons extra-virgin olive oil

1 medium acorn squash, seeded and thinly sliced or in wedges

1 pound asparagus, trimmed of woody ends and cut into 2-inch pieces

1 large shallot, thinly sliced

1 pound tilapia fillets

½ cup white wine

1 tablespoon chopped fresh flat-leaf parsley

1 teaspoon salt

¼ teaspoon freshly ground black pepper

1. Preheat the oven to 400°F. Coat a large rimmed baking sheet with the oil.

2. Arrange the squash, asparagus, and shallot in a single layer on the baking sheet. Transfer to the oven and roast until the vegetables are tender, 8 to 10 minutes.

3. Place the tilapia on top of the vegetables and add the wine.

4. Sprinkle with the parsley, salt, and pepper.

5. Return the baking sheet to the oven and roast until the tilapia is cooked through, about 15 minutes. Remove from the oven, let rest for 5 minutes, and serve.

TIPS: *If using fish that is more than ½ inch thick, the cooking time may have to be increased. Store this dish, covered, in the refrigerator for up to 48 hours. This dish does not freeze well.*

PER SERVING Calories: 246; Total Fat: 8g; Total Carbohydrates: 17g; Sugar: 2g; Fiber: 4g; Protein: 25g; Sodium: 639mg

SHRIMP-LIME BAKE WITH ZUCCHINI AND CORN

SERVES 4 / PREP TIME: 10 MINUTES / COOK TIME: 20 MINUTES

Use uncooked shelled and deveined shrimp for this dish. Leftovers can be eaten as a salad.

1 tablespoon extra-virgin olive oil

2 small zucchini, cut into ¼-inch dice

1 cup frozen corn kernels

2 scallions, both white and green parts, thinly sliced

1 teaspoon salt

½ teaspoon ground cumin

½ teaspoon chipotle chile powder

1 pound peeled shrimp, thawed if necessary

1 tablespoon finely chopped fresh cilantro

Zest and juice of 1 lime

1. Preheat the oven to 400°F. Coat a large rimmed baking sheet with the oil.

2. On the baking sheet, combine the zucchini, corn, scallions, salt, cumin, and chile powder and mix well. Arrange in a single layer.

3. Add the shrimp on top. Transfer the baking sheet to the oven and roast until the shrimp is cooked through and the vegetables are tender, 15 to 20 minutes.

4. Add the cilantro and lime zest and juice, stir to combine, and serve.

TIPS: *You can use cooked shrimp in this recipe. Follow the recipe through Step 2, and place in the oven to cook the vegetables for about 10 to 15 minutes. Add the shrimp, cilantro, and lime zest and juice, and serve. Store, covered, in the refrigerator, and eat within 48 hours.*

PER SERVING Calories: 184; Total Fat: 5g; Total Carbohydrates: 11g; Sugar: 3g; Fiber: 2g; Protein: 26g; Sodium: 846mg

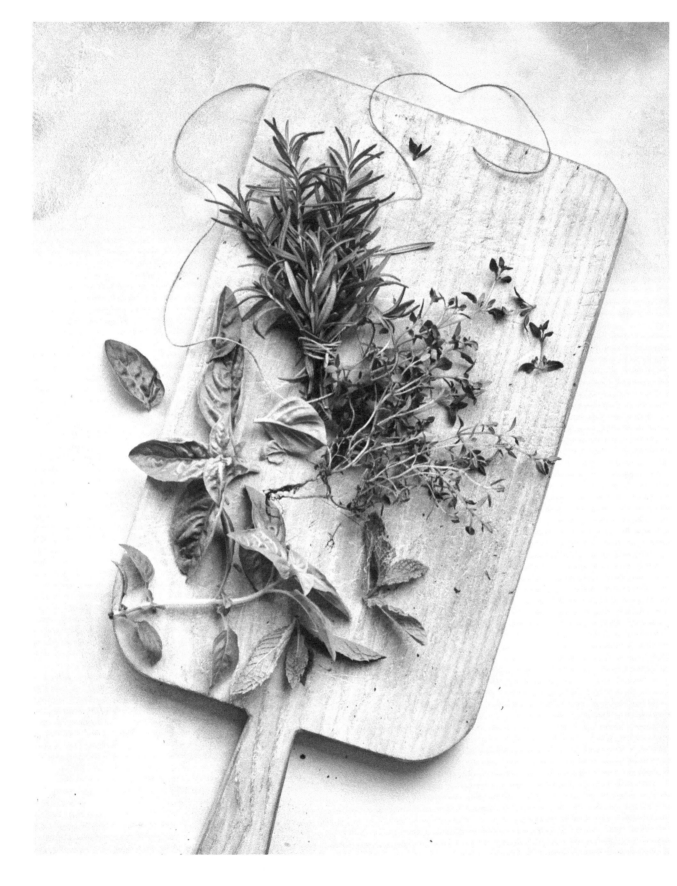

The Dirty Dozen™ and the Clean Fifteen™

A nonprofit environmental watchdog organization called Environmental Working Group (EWG) looks at data supplied by the US Department of Agriculture (USDA) and the Food and Drug Administration (FDA) about pesticide residues. Each year it compiles a list of the best and worst pesticide loads found in commercial crops. You can use these lists to decide which fruits and vegetables to buy organic to minimize your exposure to pesticides and which produce is considered safe enough to buy conventionally. This does not mean they are pesticide-free, though, so wash these fruits and vegetables thoroughly. The list is updated annually, and you can find it online at EWG.org/FoodNews.

DIRTY DOZEN™

1. strawberries
2. spinach
3. kale
4. nectarines
5. apples
6. grapes
7. peaches
8. cherries
9. pears
10. tomatoes
11. celery
12. potatoes

†Additionally, nearly three-quarters of hot pepper samples contained pesticide residues.

CLEAN FIFTEEN™

1. avocados
2. sweet corn
3. pineapples
4. sweet peas (frozen)
5. onions
6. papayas
7. eggplants
8. asparagus
9. kiwis
10. cabbages
11. cauliflower
12. cantaloupes
13. broccoli
14. mushrooms
15. honeydew melons

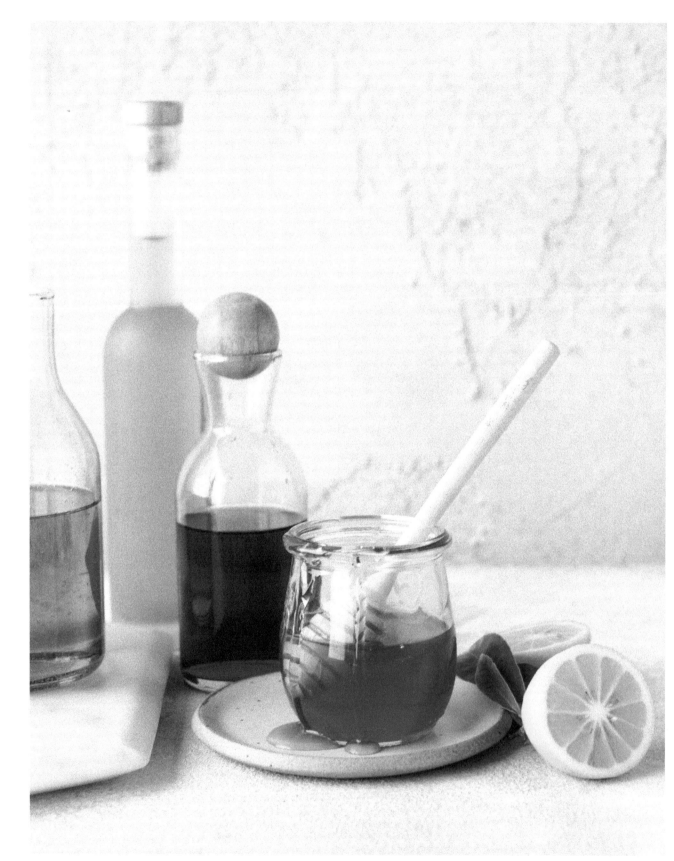

Measurement Conversions

Volume Equivalents (Liquid)

US STANDARD	US STANDARD (OUNCES)	METRIC (APPROXIMATE)
2 tablespoons	1 fl. oz.	30 mL
¼ cup	2 fl. oz.	60 mL
½ cup	4 fl. oz.	120 mL
1 cup	8 fl. oz.	240 mL
1½ cups	12 fl. oz.	355 mL
2 cups or 1 pint	16 fl. oz.	475 mL
4 cups or 1 quart	32 fl. oz.	1 L
1 gallon	128 fl. oz.	4 L

Volume Equivalents (Dry)

US STANDARD	METRIC (APPROXIMATE)
⅛ teaspoon	0.5 mL
¼ teaspoon	1 mL
½ teaspoon	2 mL
¾ teaspoon	4 mL
1 teaspoon	5 mL
1 tablespoon	15 mL
¼ cup	59 mL
⅓ cup	79 mL
½ cup	118 mL
⅔ cup	156 mL
¾ cup	177 mL
1 cup	235 mL
2 cups or 1 pint	475 mL
3 cups	700 mL
4 cups or 1 quart	1 L

Oven Temperatures

FAHRENHEIT	CELSIUS (APPROXIMATE)
250°F	120°C
300°F	150°C
325°F	165°C
350°F	180°C
375°F	190°C
400°F	200°C
425°F	220°C
450°F	230°C

Weight Equivalents

US STANDARD	METRIC (APPROXIMATE)
½ ounce	15g
1 ounce	30g
2 ounces	60g
4 ounces	115g
8 ounces	225g
12 ounces	340g
16 ounces or 1 pound	455g

Index

Acknowledgments

FROM ANA

I would like to thank my family for giving me the space to make this writing thing a reality. Also, to my supportive team of RD writers: I couldn't make it work without you.

FROM DOROTHY

I'd like to thank my friends and family, who have had to share space with my lifelong obsession with food and eating well.

I'd like also to thank my editor, Pam Kingsley, and the entire Callisto Media team, who continue to grow to create a better book.

About the Authors

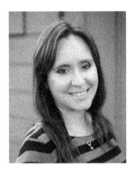

Ana Reisdorf is a registered dietitian nutritionist with 12 years of experience in the fields of nutrition and dietetics. Currently, she shares her passion for nutrition on a larger scale as a writer. She brings her clinical experience and understanding of human psychology into her writing. Ana lives in Nashville, Tennessee, with her husband and two boys. Visit her website at anareisdorf.com.

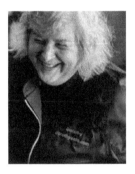

Dorothy Calimeris is a certified health coach, chef, cooking teacher, and the coauthor of *The Anti-Inflammatory Diet & Action Plans, The Good Life! Mediterranean Diet Cookbook,* and *The Complete Anti-Inflammatory Diet for Beginners*. Her passion for cooking and whole real foods is what drives her to help others transition to a healthier lifestyle by making cooking fun and easy. It's simple: We feel better when we eat better. Visit her website at dorothyeats.com.

CPSIA information can be obtained
at www.ICGtesting.com
Printed in the USA
LVHW020146160919
631152LV00001B/2/P

9 781641 528429